TABLE OF CONTENTS

CAN WE HEAL FROM CANCER?

Guy & Fred did it... And here is how

> **"May food be your medicine"**
>
> - Hippocrates

Forewords by Doctor Eric Berg and Professor Maurice Israel

Foreword #1

Once a person is diagnosed with cancer, their whole world is turned upside down, fear sets in and unfortunately this new stress alone paralyzes your immune system – the very thing that is supposed to kill cancer cells. Where do you turn? Experts? Isn't an expert someone who is expert at getting results? Apparently not when you are an expert in cancer (oncologist). The statistics on survival rates for conventional treatment of cancer is dismal. Unfortunately, doctors must follow standards of care and can't deviate. This is bad news for you because cancer is a big business and the pharmaceutical industry have a huge hand is keeping the status quo.

The stories of both Guy and Fred and others should not be downgraded to some anecdotal unscientific testimonial. Turning around stage 4 cancer to the point where there is zero cancer is a dream come true. You must realize that the survival rate for stage 4 cancer is not good. It has the highest risk of mortality. It is the most severe type of cancer. People are told to enjoy the time they have left and prepare for the worst. But Guy and Fred decided to take a different approach. This book about their story and how against all odds, they turned things around and survived. The central theme or cure they used was prolonged fasting. Something so simple, a treatment that is so inexpensive, yet so powerful that turns your immune system into a kick-ass fighting machine.

In the sea of confusion on theories about cancer, treatments for cancer, there is but one action you must include among everything else to be successful... fasting!

This book will take you by the hand and guide you showing exactly what to do.

Dr. Eric Berg

Foreword #2
Dear Guy and Fred.

How not to be moved by your respective stories, and your fight against cancer. Cancer is often created by personal histories (lifestyle or genetic) yet triggered by an intense emotional stress. I am sensitive to what happened to you, because I think of my father and many friends who went through the same disease, but who did not have your understanding of the disease, your pugnacity, and to whom a form of resignation and fatigue have sadly led to what they saw as inevitable.

Thank you for quoting me in your book along with great biochemists and doctors, like Warburg, Eigenbrodt, Mazurek, Gernez, Longo, Seyfried, and so many others who are looking for a conceptual framework to understand cancer. But I am only a retired researcher, whose specialty was not Oncology but Neurochemistry. Therefore, it is with humility and without any certainty, that I agree to write this foreword. Remember that my goal was only to understand, while yours is to help those like you who are fighting against cancer. The hypotheses that I have been able to put forward are not a validated treatment, but an experimental proposal on animal models of cancer. So please dear reader, do not put yourselves in a situation that would not be approved by oncologists, the only ones authorized to prescribe adapted treatment to patients.

Here is what I can say to simplify and summarize them for your readers.

When catabolic hormones (glucagon epinephrine, cortisol) are called upon, during fasting for example, the enzymes that ensure the production of nutrients (glucose and ketones) will be activated. To do so, protein kinases will phosphorylate and inhibit the enzymes that degrade glucose, while its production by other enzymes (neo-synthesis or glycogenolysis) will be activated. In parallel, the degradation of fatty acids into Acetyl-CoA will be triggered and the production of ketones increased. Thus, fasting mobilizes the reserves to ensure the production of glucose and ketones. Conversely, the anabolic hormones insulin secreted during a meal will promote the breakdown of glucose and the synthesis of glycogen, while the synthesis of fatty acids will block their degradation and promote the synthesis of lipids and proteins forming new membranes, for cells in mitosis. During this anabolic process, protein-phosphatases come to reverse the role of protein kinases that had been activated by catabolic hormones.

What we see in cancer is a hybrid situation. At the junction between glycolysis and oxidative metabolism, two enzymes, Pyruvate kinase and Pyruvate dehydrogenase remain blocked by phosphorylation, as if the action of catabolic hormones were maintained, while fatty acid synthesis, lipogenesis and protein synthesis is triggered by an insulin-like anabolic situation. This hybrid situation could result from an alteration of the endocrine pancreas, which normally inhibits the release of glucagon when insulin is secreted.

If glucagon=catabolism and insulin=anabolism, doesn't the hybrid situation observed during the metabolic rewiring of tumor cells deserve an attempt at "resetting" by fasting? Indeed, during fasting, Pyruvate kinase and Pyruvate dehydrogenase are inhibited by phosphorylation, and it is hoped that when this fast is interrupted, their dephosphorylation will be re-triggered, which would correct the hybrid metabolic situation of tumor cells. by this attempt to "reset" the system. It is certainly not so simple, because the ketones formed during fasting can become food for tumors. Indeed, the interruption of the last two stages of glycolysis at the start of the Krebs cycle, which explains the Warburg effect (lactic fermentation even in the presence of oxygen) indicates that the glycolytic source of Acetyl-CoA is blocked in tumor cells. But we also know that the tumor cell must necessarily manufacture these fatty acids and lipids and that this metabolic pathway (lipogenesis) automatically interrupts the fatty acid degradation pathway into Acetyl-CoA, by blocking their mitochondrial transporter. Thus, the main source of Acetyl-CoA in tumor cells will necessarily be the ketolysis of ketones, which depends on the SCOT enzyme, the product of the oxct1 gene. Blocking SCOT should then prevent the tumor from growing, during this attempt to "reset" by fasting. Blocking SCOT and ketolysis during fasting could perhaps explain the success of this metabolic reset, which at the same time avoids feeding the tumor, and would justify the regression that has been observed. It should also be added that apart from their nutritional action, ketones are also signaling molecules acting, in an extracellular position, on a receptor (HCA2), capable of inhibiting proliferation and inflammation.

So, congratulations to you both, dear Guy and Fred, because you courageously describe your journey, so that we can find the common points that have guided you during this prolonged fast, associated with supplements, which may have blocked ketolysis, upstream and downstream of SCOT.

There are certainly other observations equivalent to yours, which must be looked at with the same curiosity that allowed Dr. W. Withering in 1775 to identify Foxglove in a plant extract, used by empiricism popular, to treat heart disease.

I wish you all to continue your path to recovery, and to act in consultation with your oncologist and your attending physician.

Pr. Maurice Israel
- Former Director of Research at the CNRS (France)
- Doctor of Science, Doctor of Medicine (MD),
Doctor of Neurobiology

(Note that Professor Israel wrote more than 200 scientific publications including 20 on cancer)

Introduction

Dear reader,

This book is a synthesis of two cancer survivors' experiences (Guy Tenenbaum and Fred Evrard). It's about the path that led us to healings that were supposed to be "impossible" for Guy, and "amazing and incredibly fast" for me. This book can be seen as the second edition of our original books on cancer, but developed and enriched with our collaboration and the latest scientific research and publications, mainly the PubMed publication of the now famous SCOT study.

For better clarity, and so that you, dear reader, can compare the different protocols for yourself, some paragraphs were written jointly by the two of us, while others by Guy or Fred individually.

Please note that we are neither doctors nor biologists. As cancer survivors, and having followed quite unusual methods, we wanted to share our healing experiences and highlight the doctors and researchers who think outside the box when talking about non-toxic cancer treatments and therapies.

We do not claim to have THE solution to all cancers, and for all patients. It worked FOR US, and it is our duty to point out the path we have taken, not to convince you, but to encourage you to do your own research.

The work of Professor Thomas Seyfried, Professor Maurice Israel, Doctor Nasha Winters, Doctor Valter Longo, Doctor Henry Joyeux and many others, have been instrumental in our healings and their research has not only inspired us, but also gave us the knowledge we needed to better understand what our intuitions and common sense were telling us: Eliminate the cause and the symptoms disappear.

Neither Guy nor myself are against modern medicine, and both have used it when needed. But treating the symptoms does not replace the patient's responsibility to seek, question, investigate; nor to work on their lifestyle and stress management. Epigenetics is one of the keys to this fight and it is not in the hands of doctors, but rather in those of the patients.

We have become a pro-cancer society and our environment (internal and external) is both the cause of diseases and the key to our health. Most of what industrials sell us is carcinogenic, from the toxic processed food and food by-products, pesticides, food preservatives, antibiotics and Omega-6s in our meat, plastic particles in our water, mercury in our fish, air, water and soil pollution, stress, lack of physical activities, toxic relationships, over consumption of medical drugs, over-vaccinations, hours of sitting in front of a screen, and much more... Yes, we have become a sick and pro-cancer society. But the good news is, it is easy to make just a few changes to improve our health and our lives.

Enjoy this reading, enjoy your research and above all, enjoy a long and healthy life!

Fred Evrard and Guy Tenenbaum

PART 1: Who are Guy and Fred?

Guy and Fred are two cancer survivors who, in order to heal, have chosen to trust science rather than medicine.

Put in contact by a mutual friend, the two future friends then realized that without knowing each other or even having spoken to each other, they used almost the same protocol to heal from cancer. They met for the first time in early 2022, and have been collaborating ever since.

GUY:

The experience that I am about to share with you is the story of a long-term battle. My name is Guy Tenenbaum and I am a terminal cancer survivor. Cancer, I faced it standing up, with all my determination and a good sense of humor, despite the anxiety that never really left me. My story is that of a man who refused the prognosis, defied the statistics and who fought the disease with his own weapons.

With my story, I will show you that you can heal by combining allopathic medicine, scientific research and alternative approaches. Everything I put in place to regain my health, I did it, not because of my "beliefs", but because scientific studies attested to the results. Let's go back to the origin of the story.

I was a happy man, I had succeeded professionally, I was a fulfilled husband and father, I was leading what can be called "a good life". As a Frenchman, my daily life was made of these gourmet habits that I enjoyed so much. I liked my hot chocolate and croissant in the morning, a good high-end restaurant for lunch and dinner was an opportunity to get together with the family around a good homemade meal. The routine of millions of people! I didn't really pay attention to the contents of my plate, as long as I enjoyed myself! I was a man who fully enjoyed the pleasures of life; a "bon vivant" as we say in France...

I came to Miami 20 years ago with my wife and kids, to enjoy a well-deserved retirement. In 2018, I was diagnosed with stage 4 prostate cancer with metastases. "Incurable", the doctors said. The bones, lymphatic nodes, prostate and right side of my lung were affected. Same verdict in the USA and in France. "There's nothing that can be done...Enjoy life and the little time you have left." Same speech from

American, French and Spanish Oncologists such as "cancer always finds its way", "le cancer trouve toujours son chemin", "El cancer siempre busca su caminó". Across borders, limiting beliefs remain the same.

This is where I understood that there was a huge difference between medicine and biology and that only biologists could help me.

It was impossible for me to accept that verdict. Quite the opposite; I searched and studied, sometimes up to eighteen hours a day in order to understand and be able to act. Nobel Prize winners and some of the greatest researchers have become either my favorite authors or in some cases, my friends. Armed with that knowledge, I made it my crusade to help others through my books and videos.

FRED:

I am a French professional martial arts instructor and international speaker; I am 50 years old and have nearly forty-five years of martial arts experience. I am also a counter-terrorism consultant for the French Ministry of Defense and a close combat trainer for several elite law enforcement and special forces units in France and around the world.

In September 2020, despite a healthy lifestyle, I was diagnosed with a genetic stage 3 colon cancer, with a 10cm tumor, inoperable without dramatic consequences for my physical integrity.

Genetic predisposition (my father and my grandfather both died of cancer) and the exhaustion of my adrenal glands by repeated trips around the world were the silent root cause, but the trigger was stress. After a 4-year trip around the world and 10 years in Singapore, my wife Lila and I decided to move to the US and the (by the book) immigration process cost me a lot of time, money and emotional pressure, plus three years of waiting for and finally getting our Green Cards. Then came Covid-19, with serious professional and financial consequences for our family.

In two months, I went from the best shape of my life at 70 kg and 9% body fat, to 49 kg and being just skin and bones. That's how it all started. After the initial shock of the diagnosis (three days of self-pity, thinking I was going to die), I got up and had only three thoughts in mind:

1. I would survive this cancer
2. What doesn't kill you makes you stronger.
3. *"Let thy food be thy medicine"*

-Hippocrates

Four months later, the tumor had disappeared. I was cured. No long sessions of chemotherapy (only three sessions to manage the pain), no radiation, no surgery. Even if I still have digestive sensitivity to certain foods, the fight was basically won.

Clinique Victor Hugo
PARIS
──── VIVALTO SANTE ────

COMPTE RENDU DE COLOSCOPIE

NOM PRENOM : EVRARD, Frédéric

Né le : 13/10/1972

Date de l'examen : 10/09/2020

Anesthésiste : Dr LORENZON,

Médecin traitant : Dr

Appareil : Olympus n°10

Rappel clinique : Douleurs abdominales. Hématochésie. Contrôle endoscopique.

Rectum : lésion rectale hémi-circonférencielle antérieure ulcéro-végétante débutant à la marge anale jusqu'à 10 centimètre de celle ci.
Sigmoïde : dicerticules à collet large et fin.
Colon descendant : la muqueuse est normale.
Colon transverse : la muqueuse est normale.
L'angle droit : la muqueuse est normale
Colon ascendant : la muqueuse est normale.
Caecum : la muqueuse est normale.

CONCLUSION :

Lésion rectale.
Diverticules à collet large et fin.
Score de Boston correct (2+2+3) 7.
Temps d'exploration au retrait supérieur à 15 minutes.
Biopsies en attente.
Bilan à réaliser.

HHQE005

Dr O. SPATZIERER

Dénomination sociale : Clinique Chirurgicale Victor Hugo
5 bis, rue du Dôme - 75116 PARIS
Tél : 01 53 65 53 65 | Fax : 01 53 65 53 47
SAS au capital de 37 000€ - RCS Paris 484 112 067 - Siret 484 112 067 00022 - APE 8610Z - TVA intracommunautaire FR36484112067

www.clinique-victorhugo.fr

the oncologist in South Carolina confirmed the diagnosis
and prognosis of the French hospital

PRISMA
HEALTH.

10/15/2020

To Whom It May Concern:

Frederic Aime Evrard was in my office on 10/12/2020.He is being treated by my office
for adenocarcinoma, rectal cancer. He will be undergoing chemo and then chemo
radiation. He will possibly undergo surgery after this treatment and then continue
treatment post op. During this time he may become weak and require a care giver full
time to provide assistance in daily living activities as well as emotional support related to
cancer diagnosis and treatment.

If you have questions or concerns, please don't hesitate to call our office at
864-699-5700.

Sincerely,

████████████, MD
CANCER INSTITUTE MDC
890 W. FARIS ROAD, STE 320
GREENVILLE SC 29605-4281
864-455-1200

10/17/20 MRI Study Result
Mr. Frederic Evrard – Oct. 13, 1972

Impression

Evidence of near circumferential tumor involving the distal rectum and proximal anus with similar irregular thickening of the involved segment of the rectum.

Slice by slice comparison of the axial thin section images document more heterogeneous T2 signal intensity throughout the involved mucosal/submucosa but thickness, distribution, and contours remain similar to previous exam.

Stable mesorectal nodes.

Signed by: 10/17/2020: M█████ S██████, MD

Narrative

EXAM: MRI RECTUM WO CONTRAST, 10/17/2020

INDICATION: C20 Malignant neoplasm of rectum I10;

TECHNIQUE: Multiplanar/multisequence pelvic MRI performed without IV contrast including thin section angled axial and coronal images, oriented to the distal rectal tumor.

FINDINGS:

Distortion of the distal rectum related to treated 75% circumference tumor involving the distal rectum and proximal anus. Approximately 6 to 7 cm in length and terminates approximately 1.8 cm from the anal verge.

1/10/21 MRI Study Result
Mr. Frederic Evrard – Oct. 13, 1972

Impression

No more evidence of circumferential tumor involving the distal rectum and proximal anus

Signed by: 1/10/2021: M█████ S██████ MD

Narrative

EXAM: MRI RECTUM WO CONTRAST, 01/10/2021

INDICATION:

COMPARISON: Pelvic MRI 9/17/2020.

TECHNIQUE: Multiplanar pelvic MRI without contrast. This includes thin section angled axial and coronal images, oriented to the distal rectal tumor.

FINDINGS:

No more evidence of circumferential tumor involving the distal rectum and proximal anus. No interval local progression of disease is observed. No new adenopathy elsewhere in the pelvis.

PART 2: What is cancer?

I believe that modern medicine has it wrong. Cancer is not the disease. Cancer is the symptom; an alarm that usually follows a metabolic problem such as chronic inflammation, chronic fatigue or hyper-toxicity, some of our cellular metacondria's inability to produce energy..., and which tells us that there is too much waste in our bodies and that our immune and lymphatic systems can't fight and eliminate them properly.

Everyone develops cancer cells all the time but the body usually sheds them. Our body is designed to recognize and eliminate cells that mutate and become cancerous, and it does so very effectively if functioning properly. So, cancer isn't the problem. The problem lies in a systemic metabolic imbalance, which results in one or more tumors that grow in the body without being stopped by the immune system. The tumor is the symptom, not the cause.

The answer to cancer is not more toxins - such as months or even years of chemotherapy and radiation (which can certainly be useful in small doses, for a short period of time), but for me, those are certainly not the treatment. They simply help with the symptoms.

The answer is <u>less</u> toxins, more cleansing, lots of very high-quality micro and macro nutrients, lots of rest, stress management and helping the body to eliminate toxins via fasting, intermittent fasting, exercise, breathing, sauna, rebounding, etc.

Here is a meta-study on the long-term efficiency of chemotherapy for the treatment of cancer:

https://pubmed.ncbi.nlm.nih.gov/15630849/

Results: *The overall contribution of curative and adjuvant cytotoxic chemotherapy to over 5-year survival in adults is estimated to be 2.3% in Australia and 2.1% in the USA.*

Conclusion: *It is clear that cytotoxic chemotherapy only makes a minor contribution to cancer survival. To justify the continued funding and availability of drugs used in cytotoxic chemotherapy, a rigorous evaluation of the cost-effectiveness and impact on quality of life is urgently required.*

Is cancer psychosomatic or a metabolic disease?

Probably both. Many oncologists, like Professor Khayat in France, talk about the "psychological trigger" of cancer. If the terrain is the bullet, stress is the finger that pulls the trigger.

Guy always says it took thirty years of bad food to set the stage for his cancer, but all it took was a severe emotional shock to trigger it.

Same for Fred. Unfavorable genetics certainly didn't help but above all, several months of intense stress and his body ended up developing a cancerous tumor in order to isolate the circulating toxins.

For 50 years, cancer research was based on the hypothesis that cancer was a genetic disease. We are born with specific genes that carry the risk of developing this or that illness, and that we have no capacity for action other than heavy allopathic treatments. My first discovery concerned the work of Otto Warburg, a German doctor and chemist who received the Nobel Prize in 1931. His conclusions reveal that in most cases, the cause of cancer was not genetic but metabolic. Otto Warburg has shown that the metabolism of cancer cells differs from that of healthy cells. His observation is that the energy or lack of energy which allows the proliferation of cancer cells is generated in a different way. To supply the body with energy, a healthy cell produces ATP through the combustion of glucose and oxygen. Because the mitochondria are defective, the cancer cell uses another metabolic pathway which is none other than the fermentation of sugar.

The mitochondria is, in a way, the energy center of the cell where cellular respiration takes place and where oxygen is used for the proper functioning of the body. With this in mind, there are then two major therapeutic strategies for fighting cancer: reducing glucose on one hand and relaunching mitochondrial respiration in cells to slow down their growth on the other. Otto Warburg's research is still not accepted today (or at least not used in the care of patients).

Today, the two leaders of this thesis are Thomas Seyfried in the United States and Maurice Israel in France. Professor Seyfried is an American biochemist, professor of biology at Boston College, a graduate of the University of Illinois, who published a book about the link between cancer and metabolic dysfunction "Cancer as a Metabolic Disease".

Maurice Israël is a French professor, Doctor of Science (Paris, 1969), Doctor of Medicine (Paris 6, Pitié-Salpêtrière, 1978) and Director of the Laboratory of Cellular and Molecular Neurobiology at the CNRS (1994-2000). He has more than 200 publications to his credit.

In the idea that the dysfunction of the metabolism is the primary cause of the development of cancer, the essential action to be implemented therefore consists first of all in limiting the fermentable "fuels" of the malignant cells, mainly carbohydrates, sugars and glutamine (the most abundant amino acid in our diet), to aid in treatment. Of all the researchers I have tried to contact, they were the only two to answer.

The 2015 Nobel Prize of Medicine was given to a Chinese pharmacy researcher, Tu Youyou, who isolated the active ingredient of a plant, annual mugwort (Artemisia annua) whose medicinal properties have been known in China for more than 2000 years. This plant seems to be the most effective means we currently have to fight malaria. Henry Lai and Narendra Singh of the University of Washington demonstrated the effectiveness of this drug which could kill 98% of cancer cells, especially in blood and breast cancer. It is available in the United States but prohibited in Europe.

The 2016 Nobel Prize was given to a Japanese biologist, Yoshinori Ohsumi, who solved the mystery of autophagy by conducting experiments on yeasts.

Autophagy is a condition whereby recycling of damaged parts of the cell occurs. This includes damaged mitochondria, the exact location of where cancer is located.

He continued his work by demonstrating that the same process takes place in the human body. His discovery was going to be a pillar in our recovery. Many professors and researchers are working in this direction, such as Valter Longo (gerontologist and professor of biology at the University of Southern California) and Thomas Seyfried

The work of James Allison and Tasuku Honjo on immunotherapy and the action of the immune system on tumors (particularly T-cells) has shed additional light on the indisputable advantages of autophagy.

T-cells have the function of killing cancer cells.

Indeed, cancer cells being intelligent, they hijack our immune system to their advantage by neutralizing the T-cells supposed to defend us. (29) We discovered a wealth of information by studying the work of people such as Pr. Thomas Seyfried, Dr.

Jason Fung, Pr. David Khayat, Dr. Richard Béliveau, Pr. Henri Joyeux and of course, the videos of Dr. Eric Berg, who makes complicated information and research accessible to the public

The benefits of autophagy

The term "autophagy" was coined by 1974 Nobel Prize winner Christian de Duve.

From the Greek "auto" (oneself) and "phagein" (to eat), it literally means "to eat oneself". This natural mechanism is induced by voluntary or involuntary deprivation of food: fasting. The body is then led to produce energy by drawing from within its own biological environment. We are aware that fasting generates many controversies and fears, even though the body has always adapted to the lack of food. Since the beginning, periods of lack and deprivation have been a part of life. The body, in all the intelligence of its biology, has an alternative fuel to sugar: fat. Our love-handles are sources of stored energy, only used when food runs out. Fasting is also a practice found in all the religions of the world and which in no way constitutes a danger to the body but on the contrary, a period of rest allocated to

31

meditation, during which one refocuses on oneself, one's beliefs, one's interiority.

Fasting is also used in many traditional medicines and has been for the past 5,000 years or more!

The mechanism of autophagy comprises two phases: the catabolic phase (destruction) and the anabolic phase (reconstruction) which are the two components of metabolism (a set of chemical reactions within a living being to keep it alive and develop it). In the wrecking phase, autophagy destroys everything in the body that is unhealthy, including cancer cells. In the reconstruction phase, it repairs, clears, cleans and rebuilds. It allows the birth of new cells to replace the old ones, because they are defective or because they have been eliminated by the catabolic phase (apoptosis or natural death). To make an analogy with real estate, when a house needs to be renovated, the first thing to do is to break everything you want to change and then redraw the plans of the house. This is the catabolic phase of demolition. In the second time intervenes the anabolic phase during which one rebuilds what must be, according to the plan.

The peculiarity of cancer cells is that apoptosis does not work so they do not normally die and continue to multiply; cancer cells are almost immortal. We chose to rely first on research and then on our own experience of autophagy and we believe this is why we are still alive and thriving. To enter the state of deep autophagy that allows the body to regenerate, we first do a 36-hour to 72-hour dry fast (no food, no water) or a 5-day water fast. This is different from intermittent fasting when one does eight, fifteen or sixteen hours of fasting per day. Intermittent fasting is a method of health maintenance for people who wish to maintain a stable weight and who do not have a serious illness. This method is practiced today by millions of people around the world but when it comes to cancer, the periods of autophagy must be deeper and longer to allow the body to cleanse itself and release energy for its self-regeneration. Today, we can say without a doubt that fasting was the bedrock of our healings.

Remember that we don't <u>catch</u> cancer. We <u>develop</u> cancer, which means that it is the body itself that creates tissue in order to develop a tumor... And since the body never malfunctions and follows the universal principle of economy of energy, there must be a good reason for it.

PART 3: What do research and specialists have to say (in 2022)?

Research into a natural, side-effect-free metabolic treatment for cancer is making great progress. It is divided into several "pillars" that Guy calls the "5 essentials". Here are the 5 essentials, as used by Guy and Fred:

1st Essential: Prolonged Fasting

2nd Essential, Metabolic Treatment (as developed by Professor Maurice Israël)

The metabolic treatment protocol consists of reconciling the ketogenic diet with over-the-counter natural food supplements such as Alpha-Lipoic Acid and Garcinia Cambogia. The first is a sulfuric acid present in all cells of the body. It plays a key role in the production of energy in the body. Guy and Fred take 600mg twice a day. Alpha-Lipoic Acid acts directly at the level of the mitochondria and "recycles" all antioxidants such as vitamins E, C and glutathione. It is easily found in its natural form on the internet, without the addition of artificial products. The advantage of taking it in its natural form is that the dose to be taken is lower compared to its synthetic form, due to its high bioavailability.

One of the main sources of Alpha-Lipoic Acid is brewer's yeast. It is also found in all dark green vegetables such as kale and broccoli.

Garcinia Cambogia is a fruit grown throughout Asia, but originally from Indonesia. Hydroxycitrate is extracted from the bark of this exotic fruit. Garcinia Cambogia helps lower blood sugar, which makes it interesting for pathologies such as diabetes. It also has the advantage of suppressing sugar cravings. This treatment has no side effects but may have interactions with certain chemotherapies. Fred and Guy both use it combined with coenzyme Q10 twice a day.

Fred started this treatment, associated with high doses of melatonin (20 to 30 mg per day) under the advice of a doctor friend in France, Dr. Jean-Pierre Lablanchy. Guy started the metabolic treatment after meeting French oncologist Dr. Laurent Schwartz. Professor Maurice Israël invented the metabolic treatment twelve years ago and this protocol has been developed around the world since.

3rd Essential: Garlic

Allicin is the second element of our protocol. It is the active ingredient found in garlic but also in onions and leeks. It is a natural antibiotic that exhibits anti-cancer properties. Allicin is antioxidant, strengthens the immune system and acts in prevention against any type of disease. Guy and Fred take 2 grams in the form of supplements, twice a day, in addition to their daily consumption of fresh garlic.

4th Essential: Green tea

This powerful antioxidant is found in all green teas but in a much higher concentration in Japanese Matcha. Guy and Fred consume Matcha green tea daily throughout the day. Studies show its antioxidant, anti-inflammatory, cell-protecting and even anti-cancer properties.

5th Essential: Melatonin (a powerful SCOT's inhibitor)

Melatonin helps regulate sleep, but is also a powerful anti-cancer and antioxidant.

We take 20 mg every night for prevention and took 30 mg when we were sick. It is also possible to add phycocyanin which is one of the nutrients found in Spirulina. Again, it is antioxidant, anti-cancer, and could prevent the growth of tumors and encourage apoptosis of diseased cells. It is also one of the most efficient SCOT's inhibitors.

Updated research on the inhibition of the SCOT enzyme

If the ketogenic diet deprives cancer of its food by drastically reducing the intake of carbohydrates and sugars, Professor Maurice Israël's studies tend to show that cancer could also turn to other fuel sources to grow. Cancer could therefore use ketones (the famous Keto paradox) to manufacture acetyl coA, a process in which a metabolic enzyme called the SCOT enzyme plays a key role, since it gives cancer cells the possibility of developing by facilitating the access to emergency food.

By blocking the SCOT enzyme, which Maurice Israël considers to be "the Achilles' heel of tumors", the goal is to prevent the action of acetyl coA and glutamine which nourish cancer cells and allow them to create their membranes. Without a membrane, the cancer cell dies, weakened by the actions of Lipoic Acid, Garcinia Cambogia and the active substances that make up the protocol of our 5 essentials. Indeed, these "essentials" form a whole which is supposed to attack the SCOT enzyme itself as well as its upstream and downstream, in order to block not just an action but a whole metabolic pathway. The goal of our research is to demonstrate the effectiveness of this natural protocol which worked for us and for so many others.

Research is currently underway on derivatives of Hydroxamic Acid, including Melatonin as well as at least two other natural (and almost free) inhibitors of SCOT: Lithothamne and Phycocyanin.

This line of research is essential because it represents the potential for a natural treatment, accessible to the greatest number of people, inexpensive and non-toxic for the body.

The first promising studies have already been carried out on mice by the Nosco Pharmaceutical Laboratory, which was the first laboratory in France to seriously take into account our research on the metabolic pathway for the treatment of cancer. The results were a success since the mice to which we had administered our protocol survived in much greater numbers than those treated with chemotherapy (link to the complete study at the end of the book). The study was funded by Guy's non-profit association and Dr. Eric Berg.

We are proof that something works in this protocol. Further studies are needed to demonstrate the universal effectiveness of this protocol and pinpoint what works best and why. Among the unknowns of our study is the notion of fasting. Indeed, fasting was not taken into account in the original research on SCOT inhibition. Imagine how much more powerful the protocol will be when we start including fasting into the equation...

Today we have the chance to perhaps change the medical view on cancer treatment and help millions of people to survive this terrible disease. The method is based on natural, inexpensive and easily accessible products. Why wait? How many years, how many deaths will be necessary before the medical system opens its eyes and frees itself from the pressures of the pharmaceutical industry?

PART 4: Our full protocols

1. Fasting and autophagy

FRED:

Fasting has been proven very effective for cancer prevention and cancer treatment, for both patients under chemotherapy protocol and patients following a more natural, non-toxic treatment. Also, animal studies suggest that Intermittent Fasting might help prevent cancer.

Fasting can slow and even stop the progression of cancer, kill cancer cells, boost the immune system, and for those who choose allopathic therapies, it can significantly improve the effectiveness of chemotherapy and radiation, and reduce the side effects.

Research has been looking at calorie restriction in order to prolong and improve the quality of life for almost a century. Specifically, risk factors for atherosclerosis and diabetes are markedly reduced in humans fasting, along with inflammatory markers, like C-reactive protein (CRP) and tumor necrosis factor (TNF). Adaptation to starvation requires an organism to divert energy into multiple protective systems to minimize the damage that would reduce its effectiveness. It is thought that these systems can also prolong life and decrease cancer risk. According to a review by Dr. Longo and Dr. Fontana of the University of Southern California, calorie restriction and fasting are the most powerful and reproducible physiological interventions for increasing lifespan and protecting against cancer in mammals. Fasting reduces the levels of a number of growth factors and inflammatory cytokines, reduces oxidative stress and cell proliferation, enhances autophagy (cell destruction) and several DNA repair processes.

Read different studies here:

https://osher.ucsf.edu/patient-care/integrative-medicine-resources/cancer-and-nutrition/faq/cancer-and-fasting-calorie-restriction

https://www.ncbi.nlm.nih.gov/pmc/articles/PMC2815756/

https://stm.sciencemag.org/content/4/124/124ra27.short

https://www.ncbi.nlm.nih.gov/pubmed/22323820

https://www.ncbi.nlm.nih.gov/pubmed/3245934

I personally experienced the power of fasting for healing cancer. I used a 21-day fast in order to save my life, two of which were done at the Hippocrates

Health Institute in Florida. One of their "tools" is to feed patients raw living foods only (raw vegetables, that is, as cancer patients are not allowed sugar, therefore no fruits). But I was in such pain and so weak that I only ate the first two days, then stopped and stayed in my room pretty much the whole time. The only nutrients I ingested were coming from a glass of fresh wheatgrass juice I had once in a while. At the end of my 21-day fast, I had my second MRI... The results were impressive and against all odds, the tumor shrunk from 10cm to 6cm in length and from 13mm to 5mm in depth without any treatment other than fasting. I knew then that I was on the right path.

An article in US Health News mentions: "*Several studies suggest that fasting before chemo might alleviate common side effects like nausea and vomiting. There's also a growing body of research into whether fasting could have a beneficial effect against the cancer itself.*"

Two things happen when you fast. First, cancer cells can only feed on glucose (sugar) and glutamine (an amino-acid). Cut all sources of those two foods and you starve the tumor. Second, when fasting, the body goes into a full cleansing/elimination mode, which is the best thing you can do to remove wastes and toxins from your system. Sounds simple? Yes! But it works.

BUT if such a simple "treatment" works, why don't all the hospitals in the world use it, instead of aggressive, toxic treatments? Is it possible that it's because there is no money to make from fasting patients? I don't know... but it's a valid question, knowing that the "cancer business" is worth billions of dollars each year. I am not against "regular" treatments, and I keep my mind open to the fact that not everyone is ready to do what Guy and I did, and that not every case needs the same solution.

Fasting also helps chemo patients to better support the toxicity of the treatment. I personally fasted before two of my three chemo sessions, and I didn't get any of the side effects they told me I would get. No vomiting, no headaches, no diarrhea, no crash of the immune system (my immune system markers were all in normal range, which was a real surprise to the nurse who did my blood-work...). I didn't lose a single hair and I wasn't tired all the time. I also wanted to experiment with not fasting before one of those three sessions (the second one), and I was sick like a dog!

Using fasting along with chemotherapy is a well-known solution and several hospitals in California, Switzerland, Germany, Turkey and Russia, use fasting to control the side effects of chemo. A 3-day fast can be very effective. One day before chemo, one day during, and one more day after that. Break the fast with coconut water or vegetable juice... Done! No side effects.

One could argue that I only did three sessions of chemo and that it might be different for patients going for the full twelve to twenty-four sessions. Well, it's not. There are many testimonials from patients fasting during their full chemo treatment, who didn't have any side effects, or very little.

Here are two video links where Dr. Valter Longo (University of Southern California) talks about his study of the positive effects of fasting on the prevention and treatment of cancer:

Extreme diets and their beneficial effects during cancer treatment:

https://www.youtube.com/watch?v=1yEOJDeOM9I

Dr. Valter Longo - Fasting Cycles Retard Growth of Tumors:

https://www.youtube.com/watch?v=LGafhm1cuSI

Doctor Longo says, in the second video that *"fasting is as effective as chemotherapy"*.

Here is another video where Tomas DeLauer, a ketogenic diet and fasting expert, presents the science behind fasting to prevent or even fight cancer:

Fasting vs. Cancer Cells: Positive Science - Thomas DeLauer:

https://www.youtube.com/watch?v=WnK1FgxfIWM

Here are some of the studies he used for his video:

How fasting kills cancer cells and improves immune function. (2017, May 14):

https://www.naturalhealth365.com/fasting-cancer-cells-2238.html

Fasting-like diet turns the immune system against cancer - USC News. (2018, February 5):

https://news.usc.edu/103972/fasting-like-diet-turns-the-immune-system-against-cancer/

Intermittent Fasting for Cancer Patients Mesothelioma.net.:

https://mesothelioma.net/nutrition-and-lifestyle-for-mesothelioma-patients/

Is there a role for carbohydrate restriction in the treatment and prevention of cancer?:

https://www.ncbi.nlm.nih.gov/pmc/articles/PMC326
7662/

Last but not least, Dr. Sophia Lunt explains in her TEDx talk, how she intends to cut off cancer cells' survival potential, and describes a new way of halting their growth:

Starving cancer away | Sophia Lunt | TEDxMSU:

https://www.youtube.com/watch?v=f6rSuJ2YheQ

Unfortunately, even if there are exceptions, most doctors have no idea of the benefits of fasting on cancer treatments. Even worse, very often, for emotional support, hospital nurses give cookies and candies (pure cancer-feeding foods) as a treat to all the patients. I hope someday, medical schools will teach about health, nutrition, prevention and the human immune system...

Personally, my healing started with a 21-day fast. 21 days without any food, with water, and a small glass of fresh wheatgrass juice, from time to time (I would say about ten glasses over 21 days).

This relatively long time spent in autophagy allowed me to shrink the tumor by almost 50% in just three weeks. I knew then that I was on the right path.

GUY:

On January 19, 2019 I started a 45-day fast with a first phase of 20-day water fast, without any food and a second phase during which I took very small amounts of juice which I quickly replaced with whole raw veggies to continue to fuel my healthy cells and avoid deficiency. A distinction must be made between medical fasting in France and in other countries, such as Germany, the United States or Russia. In France, fasting most of the time implies not absorbing anything solid or liquid that would contain calories. Abroad, it is above all a matter of staying in good health and making the experience more pleasant to live in, in the best possible conditions. Professor Thomas Seyfried, during an interview, explained to me that nutrient supplementation is interesting during a fast because the body would be able to give us the necessary nutrients and vitamins for only seven days (via liver stocks). It is important to differentiate between starving cancer and undernutrition. Indeed, we see it every day with the scourge of junk food; it is possible to have a full stomach and yet be malnourished. Hunger might be satisfied but the needs of the body are not.

For those who might want to follow my example, I remind you that my practice of fasting is above all therapeutic and that it is up to everyone to carry out their own experiments, with the informed opinion of their doctors.

Fasting is not always an easy experience to go through or implement. It engages all your senses, awakens the body to lost sensations such as real hunger, sharpens the five senses and puts you face to face with your deepest emotions by the absence of palliatives such as food. The third day of fasting is a critical period, often unpleasant and well known to fasters, during which it is possible to feel a little sick. It results in symptoms such as fatigue, nausea or headaches. This moment corresponds to a phase of metabolic change during which the body, short of glucose, will feed on its lipid reserves (fat). The liver converts this fat into ketones which allow the body to feed on this alternative source of energy. After this stage, not only is vitality restored but, icing on the cake, the feeling of hunger disappears. Your body has switched fuel source and continues to function normally while engaging in the autophagy process that allows cellular regeneration.

Since the beginning of 2020, I have been continuing the fasting phases to stay in deep autophagy as often as possible, mostly to reassure myself. I admit today I'm fine but in case of relapse, I can never blame myself for not having done all that I could for my health. My method has evolved as my body has become accustomed to the practice of fasting. I have a proven technique to minimize unpleasant symptoms. At the end of the fateful three days when the body goes into ketosis, I eat a tiny amount of raw food, just enough to avoid this feeling of discomfort. For example, I can eat a small branch of broccoli or a stalk of celery, making sure not to exceed 50 calories so as not to go out of autophagy. This technique allows me to calmly live this period of fasting for 3 to 5 more days without any difficulty. I recently discovered MCT (medium chain triglyceride) oil which I sometimes take intuitively, to help me in times when I feel I have less energy. It contains fatty acids extracted from coconut, which are quickly converted into ketones. I put half a dose in my morning coffee to help my body get into ketosis faster, for a "booster" effect. Once the body is in ketosis, it should not be taken because the body will first draw its energy from oil before seeking energy from your own fat cells.

2. Intermittent fasting

Intermittent Fasting (IF) is also a powerful tool. It is an eating pattern that cycles between periods of fasting and eating. IF is based on the theory that fasting has been practiced (out of necessity) throughout human evolution and that cycling between periods of "famine" and "feasting" is an ancestrally adapted way of eating for us.

Our hunter-gatherer ancestors didn't have supermarkets, refrigerators or food available every day, year-round. Sometimes they couldn't find anything to eat for days. It is also very probable that cavemen often had to "exercise" (hunt, climb trees, run, fight...) on an empty stomach, and the improved cognitive function of fasting undoubtedly helped them to survive and find food. As a result, humans evolved to be able to function without food for extended periods of time... This educated guess made fasted-workouts very popular in many athletic circles over the past ten years.

There are many different IF protocols but here is the one we used:

OMAD (One Meal A Day): fast for 23h. Eating window is 1h.

More and more studies prove the health benefits of IF and that fasting cyclically is more natural than eating three (or more) meals a day.

I, personally, have been doing IF for almost twenty years (seriously but not religiously), simply because I feel much better doing my workout, martial arts training and HIIT, on an empty stomach.

When you fast, several things happen in your body at the cellular level; your body adjusts hormone levels to make stored body fat more accessible; your cells also initiate important repair processes and change the expression of genes.

Here are some changes that occur in your body when you fast:

- Human Growth Hormone (HGH): the levels of growth hormone skyrocket, increasing as much as five times. This has benefits for fat loss and muscle gain, to name a few.

Read the study here:

https://www.ncbi.nlm.nih.gov/pmc/articles/PMC329619/

- Insulin: insulin sensitivity improves, and the levels of insulin drop dramatically. Lower insulin levels make stored body fat more accessible for fuel. Insulin is the key to turn on/off fat deposition.

Read the study here:

https://www.ncbi.nlm.nih.gov/pubmed/15640462

- Cellular repair: when fasted, your cells initiate cellular repair processes. This includes autophagy, where cells digest and remove old and dysfunctional proteins that build up inside cells.

Read the study here:

https://www.ncbi.nlm.nih.gov/pmc/articles/PMC3106288/

- Gene expression: there are changes in the function of genes related to longevity and protection against disease and inflammation.

Read the study here:

https://www.ncbi.nlm.nih.gov/pmc/articles/PMC2622429/

These changes in hormone levels, cell function and gene expression are responsible for the health benefits of IF. Intermittent Fasting is also a powerful tool to lose weight and body fat. It boosts metabolism while helping you naturally eat fewer calories; it keeps your insulin level very low for as long as you are in a fasting period (at least half of the day or more for most people). Spending a big part of your day doing your things with zero fuel from food, you enter a state of ketosis where the body has to use its own body fat to function. If you mix IF with a Keto or low-carb diet, you will turn your body into a fat-burning-furnace.

More studies on both animals and humans have shown that IF can have powerful benefits for weight control and the health of your body and brain. It may even help you live longer.

Here are the general health benefits of Intermittent Fasting:

- Weight loss: as mentioned above, Intermittent Fasting can help you lose weight and belly fat, without having to consciously restrict calories.

- Insulin resistance: Intermittent Fasting can reduce insulin resistance, lowering blood sugar by

3–6% and dropping insulin levels by 20–31%, which could protect against type-2 diabetes

Read the study here:

https://www.sciencedirect.com/science/article/pii/S193152441400200X

- Chronic inflammation: some studies show reductions in inflammation markers, a key driver of many chronic diseases.

Read the study here:

https://www.ncbi.nlm.nih.gov/pubmed/17291990/

- Heart health: both fasting and Intermittent Fasting reduces blood triglycerides, inflammatory markers, blood sugar and insulin resistance — all risk factors for heart disease.

Read the study here:

https://www.ncbi.nlm.nih.gov/pubmed/19793855

- Cancer: animal studies suggest that IF might prevent cancer.

Read the studies here:

https://www.ncbi.nlm.nih.gov/pubmed/22323820

https://www.ncbi.nlm.nih.gov/pubmed/3245934

- Brain health: Intermittent Fasting increases the brain hormone BDNF and may aid the growth of new nerve cells. It may also protect against Alzheimer's disease.

Read the study here:

https://www.ncbi.nlm.nih.gov/pubmed/17306982

- Anti-aging: Intermittent Fasting extends the lifespan of lab rats. Studies showed that fasted rats lived 36–83% longer.

Read the study here:

https://www.karger.com/Article/Abstract/212538

For people recovering from an injury or an operation, a bone broth fast is also a very powerful tool.

3. Modified Ketogenic diet

FRED:

A Ketogenic (Keto) diet simply means to switch from using glucose to using fat for fuel.

We have a rise of obesity and cancer all around the world, and it is mainly (not only) because we eat and drink too many carbohydrates, including sugar, and consume too much processed food. By cutting down carbohydrates and increasing good fat intake, we can speed up our metabolic rate, raise our HGH (Human Growth Hormone) and Testosterone levels, and lower our insulin level so we can get healthier, balance our hormones, help regenerate our cells, build muscle and burn fat at the same time. Fat also keeps you satiated much longer than carbs, so you eat less during the day. It becomes much easier to use an Intermittent Fasting protocol.

The truth is, fat is a much better and much cleaner fuel for us than glucose (basically, fat would be the equivalent of premium unleaded fuel 98 where glucose would be diesel).

The Ketogenic diet is a very low-carb, high-fat diet, which involves drastically reducing carbohydrate intake (around 30gr. per day for men and 50gr. for women) and replacing it with healthy fats. This reduction in carbs puts our body into a metabolic state called **ketosis** (the best state for our system to fight cancer by the way). When this happens, the body becomes incredibly efficient at burning fat for energy. It also turns fat into ketones in the liver, which can supply more efficient and cleaner energy for cells, including the brain.

Ketogenic diets can cause massive reductions in blood sugar and insulin levels (another good thing to fight cancer). This, along with the increased ketones, has numerous health and fitness benefits. For this reason, more and more athletes are embracing a Keto lifestyle. Once they successfully make the switch from using carbohydrates to using fats and ketones as fuel, they find themselves leaner, healthier, and more mentally focused than ever.

There are different versions of the Ketogenic diet. Here are the ones Guy and Fred used for themselves:

FRED:

- **Modified Keto:** During cancer, my modified Keto was a moderate-fat version with approximately 55% fat instead of the common 70% (more like a high protein Keto). After the tumor was gone, I have developed my own version of the Targeted Ketogenic diet, strategically introducing root vegetable (carrots and beets) juices with a little bit of low GI fruits, on my workout days.

- Zero-carbs Ketogenic diet: This version is a high-protein and moderate-fat diet. It typically contains 40% fat, 60% protein and as close as possible to 0% carbs. This might be good for people with very high and chronic inflammation, and for people who have been poisoned by phytotoxins.

GUY:

- Modified Keto: During cancer, my modified Keto was a moderate-fat version with approximately 55% fat instead of the common 70% (more like a high protein Keto).

Foods to avoid on a Keto diet:

Any food that is high in carbohydrates should be limited. Here is a list of foods that need to be reduced or eliminated on a Keto diet:

-       **Sugary foods:** Soda, fruit juice, smoothies, cake, ice cream, candy, etc.

-       **Grains or starches:** Flour, bread, pasta, cereal, pastries, corn, rice, etc.

-       **High GI Fruits:** Low Glycemic Index fruits such as berries (strawberries, blueberries, raspberries...), grapefruits, cherries, peaches, lemon, lime are acceptable in small quantity.

-    **Beans or legumes:** Peas, peanuts, kidney beans, lentils, chickpeas, etc.

-    **Root vegetables and tubers:** Potatoes, sweet potatoes, parsnips, etc. There are a few exceptions such as beets and carrots, which are not technically Keto, but are full of anti-cancer properties, antioxidants and micro-nutrients.

-    **Low-fat or diet products:** These are highly processed and often high in carbs.

-    **Sugar-free diet foods:** These are often high in sugar alcohols, which can affect ketone levels in some cases. These foods also tend to be highly processed. Stevia and monk-fruit are OK.

-    **Some condiments or sauces:** Like ketchup or BBQ sauce... These often contain sugar and unhealthy fat.

-    **Unhealthy fats:** Try to completely eliminate processed seed oils, trans fats, margarine, industrial mayonnaise, etc.

-    **Alcohol:** Due to their carb content, many alcoholic beverages will throw you out of ketosis.

Alcohol almost acts as sugar in the body, but with even more calories per gram.

Foods to eat on a Keto diet:

You should base the majority of your meals around these foods:

-        **Fresh seasonal vegetables:** Both green and colored. In case of colon cancer where it is better not to eat too many insoluble fibers, juicing your veggies is the best option.

-        **Avocados:** Whole, ripe avocados and fresh guacamole (homemade when possible).

-        **Meat:** 100% grass-fed (aka grass-fed / grass-finished) red meat, free-range chicken and turkey (organic if possible).

-        **Fatty fish:** Such as salmon, trout, tuna and mackerel (wild-caught).

-        **Eggs:** Look for organic pastured whole eggs. Duck eggs are great also.

-        **Butter, heavy-cream and cheese:** Preferably organic and from raw milk, grass-fed and pastured animals. If you are lactose intolerant, you can use ghee. Some people think they are lactose-intolerant but the actual problem is that they respond negatively to pasteurization (which is a nutritional catastrophe) and to the synthetic hormones in "conventional" milk, and therefore, can digest organic raw milk cheeses perfectly well. Before we started pasteurizing our milk, dairy allergies were very rare because the (good) bacteria of the milk helped break down its lactose and proteins, making it easier to digest. That's why raw-milk dairy products are so much better.

-      **Extra virgin organic oils, first cold pressed**: Olive oil, coconut oil and avocado oil.

-      **Healthy oils, nuts and seeds:** Organic extra virgin olive oil, coconut oil, avocado oil, almonds, walnuts, macadamias, pecans, flax seeds...

-      **Condiments:** You can use high quality salt (which is not supposed to be white, but gray or pink), pepper and various healthy herbs and spices.

Again, it is best to base your diet primarily on fresh, whole and organic foods. They will be much better for your health and healing.

7.   Keto diet for cancer

The metabolic theory of cancer - that cancer is fueled by high carbohydrate diets - was introduced by Nobel Prize-laureate and scientist Otto Warburg in 1931. It has been largely disregarded by conventional oncology ever since, but this theory is resurging as a result of research showing incredible clinical outcomes when cancer cells are deprived of their two primary fuel sources: glucose and glutamine.

YES! Food can protect us against cancer, or be a trigger for it.

"What we have discovered is that when you try to kill a cancer cell, one of the things it does in order to survive is to spread even further. This is why chemotherapy is not the solution".

- Dr. Patrick Soon-Shiong

Here is a great video by Dr. Eric Berg on how to help fight cancer by removing glucose and blocking glutamine:

Cancer Lives on Sugar and... Something Else
https://www.youtube.com/watch?v=rewf0MMhGg8&feature=youtu.be

Doctor Thomas Seyfried's work and research on the Ketogenic diet for cancer:

- Doctor Thomas Seyfried is Professor of Biology at Boston College. He is a senior editor of the American Society of Neurochemistry's journal ASN Neuro and is on the editorial boards of Journal of Lipid Research, Neurochemical Research & Nutrition & Metabolism –

Current cancer research focuses on genetic origins of cancer, and standard treatments generally involve combinations of surgery, chemotherapy and radiation. In his book *"Cancer as Metabolic Disease"*, Pr. Thomas Seyfried presents an alternative origin of cancer based on the theories of Otto Warburg, wherein cancer is viewed as a disease of cellular metabolic dysfunction due to damaged mitochondria. In addition to pointing to new directions of research, Pr. Seyfried elaborates on a non-toxic mode of treatment, the ketogenic diet, which capitalizes on the inability of the damaged cancer cell mitochondria to metabolize ketones, thus starving them while maintaining healthy cells. Pr. Seyfried explains that since cancer cells ONLY feed on glucose and glutamine, using a primitive fermentation mechanism which doesn't include the use of oxygen, take away those two foods... and you cure cancer.

Here are two great interviews with Pr. Thomas N. Seyfried:

Interview with Thomas N. Seyfried on "Cancer as a Metabolic Disease":

https://www.youtube.com/watch?v=wY-JZ6TTNh8

Discussion on Cancer with Professor Thomas Seyfried - Dr Berg's Skype Interview:

https://www.youtube.com/watch?v=Yyt3Do4w7fs

Doctor Nasha Winters' work and research on the Ketogenic diet for cancer:

"A 2006 University of California study found that chemotherapy causes changes to the brain's metabolism and blood flow that can linger at least ten years after treatment. If cancer patients can survive conventional oncology's toxic treatment, they are far more likely to die earlier and with a lower quality of life. Leading cancer treatments such as chemotherapy and radiation are, in fact, carcinogenic, meaning they actually cause cancer long term. Indeed, many cancer drugs such as tamoxifen are classified by the International Agency for Research on Cancer (IARC) as group-1 carcinogens. So is radiation"

- Dr. Nasha Winters

When cancer patients don't obtain the desired results from conventional treatments, they come to Dr. Winters as a last hope. Because of her emphasis on whole food, nutrient-dense food, a ketogenic diet and fasting, and with adequate amount of exercise, sleep, fresh water, sunlight, love and attention, she had a very different and very effective approach to preventing and neutralizing cancer for the past 25 years, including healing her own cancer (stage 4 ovarian cancer). Her approach strays significantly from conventional oncology and has been saving many lives over the years.

A new approach to cancer is sorely needed. The long-term implications of those toxic therapies can increase gut permeability, impaired cardiovascular health, depressed cognitive and neurological functions, destroy the immune system and sometimes lead to the death of the patient.

In her book "*The metabolic approach to cancer*", she says: "*Since cancer consists of cells going awry in response to toxic diet and environments, we must optimize the body's healing mechanisms instead of waging war on them. We need to treat the terrain, not the tumor. We need to build the body up instead of attacking it. [...] When sugar, processed food, grains, soda, preservatives, additives, trans-fats, omega-6-rich oils, herbicides, pesticides and GMOs are replaced by organic vegetables and fruits, organic, 100% grass-fed meat, bone marrow and organ-meats, healthy fats and adequate hydration, the terrain shifts in a matter of days."*

Doctor Winters estimates that 90% of cancers are caused by poor, sugar-heavy diets and unhealthy lifestyles that damage mitochondrial functions.

"Cancer is not a genetic disease, as claimed by modern oncology, but instead a metabolic disorder that occurs in response to how we are feeding and treating our bodies and therefore our genomes. Through epigenetic, we have the ability to influence gene expression and mitochondrial function through our diet, lifestyle and thoughts. That's powerful medicine." she said.

Although some cancers have been proven to have a viral or bacterial origin, most of them are the result of our lifestyle, food choices and environment. Putting the patient at the core of his healing process and giving him back his responsibility for his health, rather than being a passive observer of the treatment, is the key to full and definitive recovery.

GUY:

In my fight against cancer, if I had identified autophagy as the mainstay of my healing, I could not just fast without reforming my entire lifestyle. If I wanted to survive, I had a duty to help my body in any way possible. The most obvious solution on which I had control was of course the food that I ate. I needed to put that food at the service of my health and no longer of my cancer. While eating, I had to achieve this *tour de force*: starve the disease by depriving it of its favorite fuel: sugar (all carbohydrates for that matter), while providing the energy my body needed for the fight. The industrial food that we find in our supermarkets does not match the nutritional needs of our bodies. Too processed, too refined, too sweet, too salty..., this diet makes us fat and sick because not only does it not provide the necessary nutrients, but the body must draw from its own reserves of nutrients to assimilate it. The day I met Professor Thomas Seyfried, his first question to me was "Do you know why great apes don't get cancer?" I smiled, everything was said. The great apes have no fast food or supermarkets to go shopping. They feed on what nature offers them. Of course, I have removed all industrial foods from my daily life to focus on a diet that has plenty of fresh, raw, organic vegetables and healthy proteins and fats. I had to go back to simple, essential, fresh, unpackaged, raw and living food.

The ketogenic diet was my first inspiration because it mimics fasting by limiting carbohydrates to a strict minimum, so as to force the body to feed on fat. This diet was developed in 1921 by Dr. Russel Wilder. The original medical ketogenic diet involves about 70% fat, 25% protein, and only 5% carbs. Its purpose is to limit the access of tumors to glucose and also to reduce insulin, which promotes the growth of tumor cells. It is a major asset in the fight against cancer by targeting diseased cells, as proven by multiple studies. It is in the department of Professor Thomas Seyfried, that this diet has been studied in a concrete and scientific way, especially to fight cancer. It is also increasingly requested by patients and used in addition to conventional treatments. It has the advantage of reducing the side effects of chemotherapy, increasing its effectiveness and supporting the energy and mood of patients (see Professor Valter Longo's research). Studies show very good results, particularly on brain tumors. This diet was originally given to epileptic patients but is experiencing a resurgence of interest in other neurological diseases such as Alzheimer's disease, Parkinson's disease, brain damage from strokes, diabetes and as previously mentioned, cancer. It is also recommended to have a medical or nutritional follow-up if you decide to adopt it. This diet may be a little difficult at the very beginning, until your body gets "fat adapted"). In the first days it is possible to feel fatigue, headaches, difficulty concentrating but these effects do not last. As for me, I only noticed small discomforts and dizziness during the transition to the state of ketosis. Personally, I practice a blood test each month in order to have a good visibility of the effects of my diet on my health, and to be able to adjust very quickly if necessary. Indeed, our needs evolve over time and I remain flexible in my habits, always with the idea of optimizing my routine and better nourishing my body.

Very quickly, I adapted the ketogenic diet to my lifestyle because I did not have the desire to include 70% fat in my daily diet. For protein intake, there are many choices but you always need to get the best quality you can afford, when it comes to animal products. Personally, I eat small oily fish like sardines and mackerel and eventually salmon. I do not eat larger fish because of the high concentration of heavy metals such as mercury found in the flesh of predatory species at the end of the food chain (swordfish, tuna, stingray, etc.). I stopped all grains/cereals and most of the fruits. I consume berries, making sure not to eat more than a handful a day to keep my sugar levels low while taking advantage of their antioxidant properties.

I eat antioxidant and anti-inflammatory foods daily, which allow my body to prevent oxidative stress and chronic inflammation, which are two phenomena partly responsible for the onset of a disease such as cancer. Free radicals are naturally produced by the body in the normal functioning of mitochondria, but our current lifestyles which combine a poor diet, pesticides, pollution, lack of sleep, sedentary lifestyle and stress, makes it worse. Making sure we eat a wide variety of raw and seasonal vegetables is the first key to health, supporting the body by providing antioxidants and promoting cell regeneration. Tobacco, alcohol, pasteurized dairy products, supermarket mass-produced red meat, are all pro-inflammatory and it is urgent to eliminate them from our daily lives and leave plenty of room for organic plants rich in micronutrients and first-class animal products rich in Omega-3 which, through their anti-inflammatory actions will strengthen your immune system and help fight cancer.

Today, if my pain has disappeared, it's because I have no or very little inflammation in my body.

Through my natural and physiologically adapted diet, I help my body to heal.

4. Natural supplements (in the form of "super foods" or pills)

GUY:

A. My superfoods

Matcha green tea, the drink of the Samurai

Green tea contains epigallocatechin gallates (EGCG) which is the main catechin, a polyphenol whose antioxidant action is very powerful. A Japanese study carried out on a large number of patients showed that EGCG limits the growth of malignant cells as well as the growth of the vessels that feed them in the context of prostate cancer. On the other hand, it would prevent diseased cells from absorbing the glutamine they feed on. I mix my powdered green tea with sparkling water and mint which I drink throughout the day. I chose Japanese green tea because it has 137 times more EGCG than regular green tea, making it one of the strongest antioxidants in the world. The samurai drank this tea before going into battle for its invigorating properties on body and mind. I add ginger, turmeric, chili and black pepper.

Bell Pepper

It is antioxidant, anti-aging and anti-cancer. Bell pepper is a true ally of longevity. Studies conducted on its composition show that it contains a lot of vitamin C: up to 150 mg per 100g, almost as much as parsley and twice as much as orange or kiwi. It is therefore excellent for stimulating the body's defenses. As vitamin C has major antioxidant properties, peppers also effectively fight against free radicals and premature aging. It is therefore a brake against malignant cells. Thanks to its richness in vitamin C, bell pepper combines specifically anti-cancer molecules (flavonoids, capsiates) capable of preventing but also slowing down the development of cancer cells, and even leading them to apoptosis (programmed cell death). Like green tea, it also has the ability to prevent their absorption of glutamine. For my part, I generally eat green bell peppers because they are the least sweet.

Red: the pepper is ripe, this is when it is richest in vitamin C, but also in vitamin B6 and E as well as in beta-carotene and lycopene, antioxidant pigments.

Yellow: the growth of the pepper is halfway through, this is where it is the mildest in taste, the sweetest. It is particularly rich in beta-carotene and flavonoids, but also in vitamin B9.

Green: the pepper is picked at the beginning of its growth. It contains the most flavonoids, the content of which gradually decreases as the pepper ripens. It is also a source of vitamin K.

Cruciferous vegetables

The cruciferous family includes green cabbage, red cabbage, kale (kale), broccoli, Chinese cabbage, Brussels sprouts and cauliflower. Because of their high concentration of glucosinolates and isothiocyanates, these vegetables are antifungal, antibacterial and anticancer. They would block the proliferation of cancerous cells, intervene in the death of diseased cells and prevent metastases. Finally, the indoles (chemical compounds) of crucifers inhibit the activity of estrogen receptors, which makes them serious candidates for the prevention of breast and prostate cancers. I mostly eat kale, cauliflower, broccoli (often young sprouts that contain ten times more antioxidants than mature broccoli), green cabbage, Chinese cabbage, and Brussels sprouts. I eat them raw with a sugar-free hot sauce or avocado oil mayonnaise.

Garlic

This aromatic plant is the Rolls Royce of antioxidants. It is used worldwide to treat and prevent disease. Hippocrates, father of medicine, recommended its consumption in large quantities and considered the plant as a remedy in its own right.

A study conducted in China reveals that regularly consuming raw garlic can reduce the risk of lung cancer by half and previous studies have already suggested that it may also act against other malignancies, such as colon cancer.

For better action of the garlic, it is recommended to crush the cloves, without removing the germ and to let them rest for at least fifteen minutes before eating them. This time is needed to release the enzyme called allicin. It is what produces the antifungal and anti-cancer compounds that make garlic so valuable in healthy eating. Alliaceans (garlic, onion, chives) and their cousins (leek, shallot) improve liver detoxification and thereby help protect our genes from mutations. I consume it daily: I eat the fresh cloves; I take garlic capsules and I sprinkle my dishes with dehydrated garlic powder. I put it in everything I eat because it is the anti-cancer food par excellence.

Omega-3

Omega-3, like omega-6, are essential fatty acids that the body cannot manufacture on its own and which must therefore be provided by food. I consume my omega-3s in fish like mackerel, sardines and herring or anchovies.

There are some organic eggs on the market enriched with omega-3 by adding flaxseed to the hen's diet, it is an interesting contribution. My plant sources of omega-3s are chia seeds, flax seeds, avocados, almonds, olive and avocado oil. Omega-3s have an anti-inflammatory action and protect the cardiovascular system.

For good health, it is recommended to avoid omega-6s as much as possible, which are pro-inflammatory. It is found everywhere in food. The excess is therefore more to be monitored than the risk of deficiency. I supplement as much as possible with omega-3s and avoid omega-6s as much as possible.

"Omega 3 DHA 500mg + EPA 250mg can help kill tumor cells, especially if consumed during a water fast. We believe that this mechanism involves the action of reactive oxygen species (ROS). DHA and EPA would enter the cancer cell membranes, be attacked by ROS and thus kill the cancer cell by damaging the cancer cell membranes."

- Professor Maurice Israël

Turmeric and Ginger

Turmeric and ginger are two Asian spices with recognized anti-inflammatory and antioxidant properties. Curcumin is the molecule that gives turmeric its yellow color. Known as the spice of long life, it has always been used in Ayurvedic, Chinese and Japanese medicine for its healing properties. To make the molecule more assimilable and intensify its active ingredients, we recommend combining it with olive oil and black pepper. Curcumin has been identified as an asset in the fight against cancer because studies show that it is toxic to cancer cells, promoting apoptosis. It is noted that in India where turmeric is consumed daily in dishes, cases of prostate cancer are very rare.

Ginger is also a powerful antioxidant. The gingerol it contains has well-known anti-inflammatory and anti-cancer properties that have been demonstrated in vitro. Moreover, a recent study demonstrated a promising effect as a therapeutic agent in the treatment of prostate cancer. I consume them fresh, in powder and in tablets every day.

Pomegranate

Highly concentrated in antioxidants, the juice and the skin of the pomegranate would have "an action three to four times greater than that of red wine or green tea", writes David Khayat, oncologist, Professor and head of the Oncology department at the Pitié-Salpêtrière Hospital President of AVEC, Association for Life – Hope against Cancer.

According to him, the pomegranate is "one of the most powerful cancer-preventing dietary agents". For men, it would slow down prostate cancer cells, and for women, it would have beneficial effects on certain breast cancers. I consume it in capsules morning and evening and rarely the fruit because it contains a lot of sugar.

Dark chocolate and raw cacao

Consumed in moderation, dark chocolate (minimum 90% cocoa) is recognized as anti-cancer thanks to its flavonoids. A single square of dark chocolate contains twice as many polyphenols as a glass of red wine and almost as much as a cup of long-brewed green tea. Studies have shown that dark chocolate delays the development of certain cancers such as lung cancer. I only consume 100% cocoa in squares or powder.

B. My supplements

Supplementation has been an integral part of my daily life since the announcement of cancer. I consume about thirty food supplements each day that I spread over the day. For better absorption, I consume my vitamins in the morning and the minerals in the evening since Cancer develops at night. (Weizmann Institute 2014). Due to the lack of therapeutic studies on dietary supplements, I cannot know what exactly works for me for my cancer.

To put the odds on my side, I have therefore drawn up a list of supplements that I take first because the food we eat today contains far fewer micronutrients than 50 years ago and especially that I eat very little and little variety. This supplementation also allows me to fast very regularly without worrying about drawing on my vitamin and mineral reserves and risking deficiencies. I adjust the products and the doses according to the results of my blood tests.

What matters to me is the observation that the protocol I take every day seems to be working on me. The studies do not make it possible to know whether all of these mixed supplements present interactions with each other or not.

Do not supplement without the advice of your doctors. The following list is not a magic recipe, although I readily admit playing the sorcerer's apprentice. These products are the result of my personal research and represent only a part of all the actions that allowed me to get out of it. However, I hope that one day, through research, we will be able to determine what works in cancer therapy.

Vitamins:

Group B vitamins are best taken as a complex of vitamins of the same group such as B3 and B2. They prevent me from deficiencies during my fasting phases.

Vitamin B12 is to be taken only in the event of a deficiency because the body makes reserves of it. Some articles explain that it can promote cancer in case of excess. As with iron, care must be taken not to exceed the recommended levels. It is mainly found in meats and animal products. As I do not consume them, I supplement myself to prevent any risk of anemia and limit the tremors of my hand.

Too much vitamin A can be toxic to the liver. So, I do regular blood tests to know where I am.

Vitamin D3 tablet is a marvel that strengthens the immune system, it strengthens the bones because it helps to fix calcium, associated with vitamin K2 MK7. The ampoules that we are prescribed every 3 months include doses too large to be absorbed. It is more interesting to supplement daily, in pill, to absorb the right dose. It is a liposoluble vitamin (soluble in fats) that is interesting to take during the meal, at the same time for example as a fatty fish or an avocado, source of good fat, to better fix it and absorb. Weather permitting, simply sunbathe for a while each day, being careful not to blush your skin. The sun is the most pleasant natural source of vitamin D. I live in Florida where the weather is very sunny, which allows me to enjoy the benefits of the sun every day.

Vitamin E is an antioxidant. It is preferable to take it in the tocotrienol form which is more difficult to find rather than the tocopherol form because it penetrates the cells more easily, which accentuates its antioxidant power.

Vitamin C, like vitamin D, is essential. As with any product, whenever possible, it is best to take it in its natural form: acerola rosehip. The dose of vitamin C will be lower in rosehip but it is accompanied by polyphenols and flavonoids which are as antioxidant as vitamin C, which is a plus. Combined with alpha lipoic acid, the blend recycles all of the antioxidants in your body.

Minerals:

Potassium, like vitamin A and iron, should only be taken if your blood test reveals a deficiency and never without the agreement of your doctor. It is interesting to take it during the long fast. It is found in particular in bananas which are too sweet to be part of my anti-cancer diet.

Magnesium energizes the body and increases immune defenses. It helps to fight against fatigue and avoids the phenomena of cramps. Muscle cramps and twitches are also a way of knowing that you are deficient. Magnesium also improves morale through its regulatory action on the nervous system. The best form is bisglycinate combined with magnesium citrate and taurine. It is well tolerated on the digestive plan and is better assimilated than the other forms. Beware of marine magnesium which is fashionable in drugstores but unfortunately not easily assimilated by the body. The same goes for magnesium chloride, which can attack the digestive tract and cause diarrhea, just like pidolate. Combined with vitamin B6, magnesium is better absorbed.

Zinc is an excellent immune defense stimulant. For better absorption, I prefer zinc orotate. As with any product, I do not abuse dosages which can be dangerous in the long term. To stay within the health norm, you should never exceed 50 mg of zinc per day.

Selenium is an antioxidant that cleanses the body.

Enzymes:

Coenzyme Q10 is essential for waking up the mitochondria which produce energy in our cells and prevent dental loosening.

Bromelain is an enzyme that helps digest proteins, which is interesting in the context of cancer because it allows allopathic treatments to attack tumors more easily.

Plant Extracts:

Garcinia Cambogia limits blood sugar and helps fight diabetes. It would have an anti-cancer effect.

Quercetin has anti-inflammatory and antioxidant properties. It is found in the onion. It is also excellent for the health of the intestines.

The pomegranate is interesting in the context of cancer and protects the heart. Taking it as a tablet avoids the sugar in the fruit.
Turmeric is part of my daily cocktail, which I mix with my matcha green tea with black pepper, cinnamon, ginger and cayenne pepper, at the rate of about 2 liters a day.

Echinacea is an immune defense stimulating plant that can be found very easily in drugstores, organic stores and on the internet.

Ginger: I take it in powder rather than in root to benefit from a larger dose of active ingredients.

Propolis: stimulating the immune system, it is also a natural antibiotic. Studies highlight its antioxidant and anti-cancer properties.

Other:

Honey: I take it with caution because it is sugar. I eat a small teaspoon of it in case of hypoglycemia. The sugar in honey, it is said, does not have the same impact on cancer as other carbohydrates.

FRED

A. My superfoods

Anti-cancer, anti-angiogenic, and DNA-protecting and repairing foods

- Sprouted Broccoli Seeds
- Sauerkraut (lactofermented raw cabbage)
- Organic and raw walnuts
- Garlic
- Berries (blueberries, blackberries, strawberries, raspberries...)
- Raw Cocoa
- Matcha green tea

- Olive oil
- Kale
- Pak Choy
- Parsley
- Turmeric
- Caviar/salmon roe/salmon (wild)
- Beet juice
- Celery
- Collagen
- Cooked peeled tomatoes (tomato sauce without added sugar)
- Bone Broth
- Meats and organs (organic and from free-range, grass-fed animals for herbivores)
- In low doses: raw Manuka honey

Foods That Boost Stem Cell Reproduction

- Berries (blueberries, blackberries, strawberries, raspberries...)
- Cocoa
- Green tea
- Spinach
- Kale
- Turmeric
- Caviar/salmon roe/salmon/seafood (wild)

Foods That Destroy Cancer Stem Cells

- Raw Cocoa
- Green tea
- Celery
- Carrots

   B. My supplements

- Vitamin D3 30,000 ui + K2 300
- Zinc: 30 mg
- Omega 3 + DHA 500
- EPA 250: 1000 mg
- Alpha Lipoic Acid: 1800 mg
- Garcinia Cambogia: 3200 mg
- COQ10: 300mg (x3)
- Garlic: 2400 mg
- Melatonin: 30 mg
- Quercetin: 1000 mg (1x2)
- Bromelain (3600 gdu): 1000 mg (1x2)

   5. SCOT's inhibitors

We have already extensively discussed the inhibition of SCOT in the chapter on "research in

2022", but we wanted to "add a layer" because it is, according to us (who are not doctors but experimenters), one of the main keys, along with prolonged fasting, to our healing.

In allopathic medicine, many treatments are used without long-term visibility of their side effects. Why not enrich it with non-toxic natural treatments? Melatonin, for example, between 20 mg to 30 mg per day, causes cancer to regress, maybe even disappear. Time after time, researchers have observed it without knowing why. Research is ongoing and just like Lithostat, Melatonin is a derivative of Hydroxamic Acid therefore an inhibitor of the SCOT enzyme just like Pimozide adopted by the FDA. This is (most certainly) why it is so effective in the treatment of cancer.

But it is also completely ignored by modern medicine and the big pharmaceutical companies! So much so that in France, you cannot get Melatonin at more than 1.9mg; 5mg if you are a doctor or have a prescription, whereas in the United States, it is easily found at 20mg on Amazon.com, Crazy! Especially since it has zero side effects.

But hey... business is business and Big Pharma is watching.

6. Mental strength

Famous psychologist and psychotherapist, Anne Ancelin Schützenberger, best known for her research in the field of psycho-genealogy, supports the virtues of optimism in the healing process of cancer. She explains to us:

"We have a very particular psychosomatic functioning. [...] It is critical to teach people that good mood and the will to live play a key role in surviving cancer. It seems important to me to give back to people, and especially to cancer patients, the taste for life."

We can only agree with this speech, and we have both experienced the importance of mental strength in our healing process. Have the willpower to fast for 21 days, which is not easy; firmly believing that healing is not only possible, but already there, within reach. All of this is essential.

We both agree that faith in our body's healing ability is the main reason we are still alive. He who resigns himself and accepts the prognosis of the doctors is already dead.

7. Physical activity and HIIT

Exercise, and especially fasted exercise (on an empty stomach), speeds up the elimination and cleansing process of the body, and that is why it is one of the tools we have used to survive.

Here's a great article on how exercise can help prevent or fight cancer:

https://www.the-scientist.com/features/regular-exercise-helps-patients-combat-cancer-67317

The advantage of HIIT (High Intensity Interval training, a short high intensity workout) is that it is very effective, does not last long (1 round = 4 minutes), and produces doses of lactic acids well less than "classic" training sessions lasting an hour or more. By adding stretching and walking, lactic acid elimination and recovery are optimal, which of course is beneficial in helping the body fight cancer.

7. Sun exposure

Since 1992, exposure to the sun has been classified as carcinogenic by the IARC... Whereas since the dawn of humanity, the latter has accompanied us without the slightest concern; whereas it has always NOURISHED LIFE!

Would the sun have changed since 1992? These ridiculous shortcuts, without taking into account our own poor health, really makes us laugh. Wouldn't it be our way of life, our food, our stress, our lack of sleep, our metabolic weakness and our inability to manage natural external pressure (sun, heat, cold, hunger...) that have changed rather than THE SUN???

When it is too hot, in summer we complain; but if it's cold and it's raining, we're unhappy.

When it is too cold, in winter we complain; but if it doesn't snow on Christmas, we're unhappy.

At the beach, we either slather on carcinogenic sunscreen, or let yourself get burned between noon and 2pm, while stuffing yourself with donuts, ice cream and coke...

Almost all of us want to lose weight, but most of us can't even consider skipping a meal. Or cut down on sugar. And when we have eaten too much, we complain...

Let's be a bit logical. Has the sun suddenly become our enemy, or does our current way of life no longer make sense to our biology?

We need to remember to get outside, play in the sun and reconnect with nature. Direct exposure to sunlight and UV promotes the synthesis of vitamin D and nitric oxide in the skin. This helps regulate hormones, lower blood pressure and increase blood flow throughout the body. Daily exposure of our skin to the sun can also help our body enter its natural circadian rhythm cycle which promotes sleep, recovery and muscle growth (crucial for anyone dealing with cancer).

There is no doubt for us today that direct (but reasonable) sun exposure is strongly anti-cancer, mainly, but not only, because of vitamin D3 and the production of melatonin. Here is a study that clearly explains how regular exposure to the sun reduces the risk of colon cancer:

8. Cold exposure (Cryotherapy) and hormesis

"What doesn't kill us makes us stronger"

- Nietzsche

This quote is close to the very definition of the law of hormesis: Any organism exposed to an intense but brief stress will see its functions improve. This amazing principle, shared by all living beings, is one of the essential axes for strengthening one's health and having a stronger and more resistant body, mind and spirit.

FRED

Cryotherapy uses extreme cold to strengthen the immune system and, in some cases, destroy cancer cells. In those cases, during cryotherapy treatment, the doctor freezes the cancer cells to kill them. Cold strengthening can be used different ways and via three possible vectors: in a cryotherapy chamber, in water or via the air:

1. In a chamber where the temperature drops to −110°C through the injection of nitrogen air (1 to 3 minutes)

2. Extreme cold in water at -5°C for a short time (30 seconds to 2 minutes)

3. Moderate cold by air for longer periods (20 to 30 minutes outside at 0°C

Read a few studies on the subject:

Cancer Cryotherapy: Evolution and Biology:

https://www.ncbi.nlm.nih.gov/pmc/articles/PMC1472868/

Exposure to extreme cold can also help cancer patients by reducing inflammation, as shown in this study:

https://www.ncbi.nlm.nih.gov/pmc/articles/PMC5411446

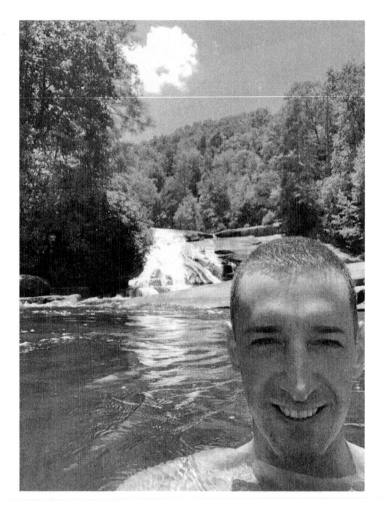

Exposure to cold to boost the immune system in mountain waterfalls (water at 3°)

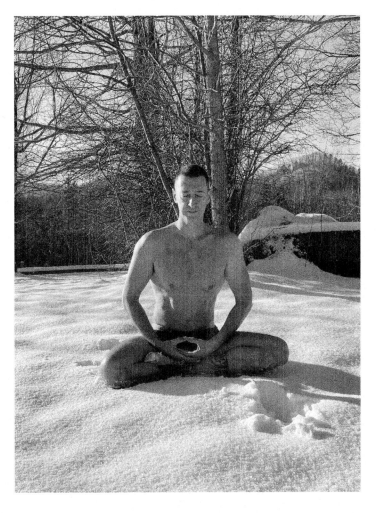

15 minutes of meditation at -3° in the snow

9. Mini-trampoline (rebounding)

-   Rebounding stimulates lymph circulation – a very good thing for healing cancer

Lymph starts its life as plasma in arterial blood. When the blood filters through tissue to deliver nutrients to cells and remove waste products, not all of it returns to the circulatory system. The 10% or so that is left behind becomes lymph and moves through the lymphatic system up towards the neck before it's dumped back into the bloodstream at the subclavian veins. Along the way it gets filtered by the lymph nodes and any nasties are attacked by white blood cells. According to the Ehrlich Lymph Organization, "*Lymph nodes also trap and destroy cancer cells to slow the spread of cancer until they are overwhelmed by it.*"

Having a highly functioning lymphatic system is essential for your overall health and ability to fight cancer. The lymphatic system is comprised of several organs including the spleen, tonsils and lymph nodes, which are interconnected by a web of fine lymphatic vessels. The lymphatic system receives toxins and metabolic waste which are transported by the lymphatic fluid to the lymph nodes, to be discharged to the kidneys and liver for elimination. So, without the lymphatic system, the body cannot effectively remove toxins.

The body has three times as much lymph as it does blood. But whereas the circulatory system has the heart to pump blood through the body, the lymphatic system depends purely on the movement of muscles and joints to move that fluid around. The rebounding action of a mini-trampoline is especially effective at moving lymph towards the nodes on its way to being filtered and detoxified. The flow of lymph is controlled by one-way valves that prevent backflow. In the absence of a pump, the motion of the rebounder helps coordinate the opening and closing of those valves so things move along nicely.

- Rebounding boosts the immune system – another very good thing for healing cancer

Circulating lymph makes it easier for the immune system to eliminate all the wastes and toxins. Not only does healthy lymph movement push waste towards lymph nodes for processing, jumping on a mini-trampoline activates human lymphocytes (specialized white blood cells which research suggests can kill tumor cells). In fact, these are the same white blood cells that are leveraged by some immunotherapy protocols. After only two minutes of jumping on a trampoline the number of white blood cells triples and remains elevated for up to an hour.

- Rebounding increases oxygen intake – again, a very good thing for healing cancer

As we saw before, cancer cells are anaerobic and thrive in a low oxygen environment and in fact cannot survive in an oxygen-rich environment as evidenced by a 2000 study published in Cancer Research Journal among many other studies. One important tool as we "tend the soil" of our bodies to create a cancer-hostile environment by saturating our tissues with oxygen.

10. Surroundings and environment

FRED

It may seem obvious, but having the unconditional support of your loved ones is essential in the healing process. I am extremely lucky that my wife, my family and all my close friends had complete confidence in me and in my way of thinking. Not once was I told I was crazy, or even urged to opt for a "classic" allopathic treatment.

My wife Lila in particular has been absolutely amazing in these difficult times. She took care of all my martial arts classes, had to take a part-time job because all our companies were on "stand-by" because of Covid-19 (or rather because of the way this crisis was stupidly managed... High doses of vitamin C and vitamin D3, and we were talking about it! Anyway...), she took care of me, supported me, took care of the house, the dog and did not ever complain. She only cried once during those four months, and that was the day I called her from France to tell her I had cancer. What an exceptional warrior.

My mom was also amazing and supported every decision I made. She was there for me like only a mother can be, and was a big part of my recovery as well.

11. Guy and Fred's daily protocols and routines

GUY:

My special anti-cancer ketogenic diet – the list of my daily foods

- Unsweetened and raw vegetables (garlic, onion, crucifers, green pepper, asparagus, mushrooms, celery, spring onion, etc.)

- No fruits except berries and lemon
- Small fish (sardines, mackerel, anchovies, etc.)
- Shrimp, eggs
- poultry, turkey, pork (on exception)
- The lawyers
- The olives
- Olive oil and avocado oil, almonds, Brazil nuts and chia and flax seeds
- Mayonnaise with avocado or olive oil and hot sauce without sugar, mustard, cider vinegar
- Spices (turmeric, cinnamon, ginger, etc.)
- Aromatic herbs (parsley, oregano, basil, mint etc.)
- From time to time, dark chocolate with a minimum of 90% cocoa and unsweetened cocoa powder
- Coffee without sugar, almond milk and matcha and mint green tea
- No conventional mass-produced red meat (too rich in Omega-6 and too inflammatory)
- No dairy products or cheese (lactose and casein in these products do not fit into my diet)

My typical daily meal consists of a plate of raw vegetables that I vary from day to day:

- 1 green salad
- 1 raw onion
- Raw broccoli / cauliflower
- Raw celery
- 1 bell pepper
- 1 avocado
- 3 cloves of garlic
- Hummus to dip my raw vegetables
- Turmeric, ginger
- Fatty fish in olive oil (usually sardines or salmon)

My sauces and condiments:

Crudités alone can seem a bit bland and monotonous. To bring taste and vary the flavors, I use accompaniments and sauces.

- Simple mayonnaise to which I very often add 3 cloves of fresh pressed garlic, to combine business with pleasure
- Dijon mustard mixed with a little apple cider vinegar
- Hummus

- Commercial sauces without sugar or preservatives

I am very attentive to the ingredients contained in sauces such as additives, carbohydrates or sugar. Read labels carefully before buying anything and always prefer fresh, unprocessed produce. I systematically check the absence of nitrates, nitrites, pesticides, carbohydrates, anything that ends in "...ose" and which are hidden sugars, as well as all preservatives. It is often better to buy less and eat as you go than to buy large volumes that contain a lot of preservatives and chemical additives.

FRED:

6am: Intermittent Fasting until 2pm (dry fast)
Cold exposure #1: 20min. outside in my underwear at 0°C (32°F)

7am: Meditation / deep breathing / Tai Chi

9am: HIIT 3 to 4 times a week (after the tumor was gone) / 3min. of mini-trampoline everyday

10am:
-   Cold exposure #2: Ice-cold bath to boost the immune system and reduce inflammation. I

do mine in mountain waterfalls 3 times a week and in the shower (not as cold) the rest of the time)
- Once a week: Psychotherapy
- Once every two weeks: Full body massage
- Once a month: Chiropractic session

12pm: Workout (weight lifting or CrossFit) 4 times a week (45min. sessions), after the tumor was gone.

2pm: I break my fast with a fresh vegetable juice (made with organic, seasonal, fresh and local vegetables) and broccoli sprouts
+ Vit D3: 20,000 iu with 200 mcg of vit. K2
+ Vit C: 4 gr
+ Turmeric: 1 tsp
+ Zinc: 30 mg
+ Omega 3 (fish oil): 1000 mg + DHA 500

3pm: Wheatgrass juice mixed with Matcha tea

4pm: Ketogenic meal: usually organic, 100% grass-fed ribeye steak + garlic + olive oil
+ Vit D3: 10,000 iu with 100 mcg of vit. K2
+ Vit C: 2 gr
+ Turmeric: 1 tsp
+ Digestive enzymes
+ Bromelain: 1000 mg
+ Alpha Lipoic Acid: 1200 mg
+ Garcinia Cambogia: 3200 mg

4:30pm: Macha green tea (just after red meat to minimize the absorption of glutamine)
+ 30 mg of melatonin

Start Intermittent Fasting until 2pm the next day

9:30pm: Bed time

PART 5: After cancer

1. Dealing with fear

Despite our victories over cancer, we are not yet "out of the woods."

We want more than healing... We want full health, physical and emotional because, while getting rid of a tumor is relatively easy, getting rid of the fear of it coming back is another story.

Without falling into paranoia or anxiety, you have to (re)motivate yourself every day, stay centered, focused, positive, disciplined, while keeping a certain lightness, pleasure, joy, recognition and of course, of sharing.

We take advantage of this chapter to thank all the people who supported us, and still support us, because if life was complicated and difficult during this "adventure", it was just as much our companions; these exceptional women, and for our families, our friends. Thank you to all of you.

2. Dealing with stress

GUY:

After the diagnosis, I had to make decisive choices to survive. I already knew that I had prepared the terrain for that cancer for the past fifty years by mistreating my body, but what was the trigger for this cancer was an intimate wound that gnawed at me from inside. For three years I didn't sleep; I was tortured by a family history that never left my head. It was the source of intense stress that I carried within my body and which weighed heavily on my heart. When I decided to fight for my life, I chose to be my main source of focus. I made an effort to remove all stress from my life. If I had been my worst enemy by bullying myself unconsciously, I had to make the decision to finally make peace with myself and stop thinking about my family burdens.

Hundreds of articles link a sudden traumatic event to the onset of cancer. Each first appointment with an oncologist, he always asked me the same question: "did you recently suffer a shock, a trauma, a loss, a divorce or any other painful event?" Stress leads to an increase of cortisol, which is a disease factor if the source of stress becomes chronic. Professor. David Khayat, a French oncologist and former head of the oncology department at Pitié Salpêtrière, has written an excellent book on that subject.

I made a list of everything that was detrimental to my well-being. I first put aside my family wounds, I got out of this toxic framework to think about myself and focus on my healing.

My work in real estate also subjected me to a lot of stress. I decided to stop working and let my son and my daughter take over the business. I got out of this stressful professional life. I needed time, a lot of time to face this cancer and I had no intention of giving in to it. Today I continue to watch over my business but from afar, and I refrain from taking on any fight other than cancer research. I now choose the fights that motivate me and make me feel alive. If cancer weakens the body, the mind remains our best ally; as long as there is still a possibility to make decisions, it is never too late. I made a conscious choice to free myself, to go beyond my deepest sorrows, to let go of whatever I didn't need to fight and heal. I faced doubt, fears of the future, the anxiety of disappearing, but I didn't surrender. I took a firm position - first in my head, I put myself in a position of mental strength: "No, I'm not going to die. Yes, I'm going to live." I've lost count of the number of times I've woken up at night crying and said to myself "one morning I'm going to wake up dead."

I thought of my family, of everything that is dear to me. I chose my destiny, made room in my life for healing, because it is in one's head that everything begins and that everything ends.

3. Sugar

GUY:

Do we need sugar? The answer is no because the body knows how to create energy from different sources such as fat for example. Sugar, starches, potatoes, refined sugars, candies, etc. raise insulin levels: the storage hormone that makes us fat. By consuming these high sugar products, insulin resistance occurs. Proteins also raise insulin, but to a lesser extent. Fats on the other hand, do not cause such a rise. This is where deep autophagy can begin.

Hunger, sugar cravings, unstable blood sugar (very high/very low), fatigue and many illnesses are linked to high insulin levels. Many studies have proven that sugar is like a drug and feeds cancer.

Artificial sweetener trap

Sweeteners feed the taste for sugar and raise insulin in the same way as real sugar, with a few exceptions. These products, even natural ones like stevia or agave syrup, are of no interest to me because they maintain a form of addiction. To avoid stimulating my appetite for sweets, I prefer to discard these products which are ultra-processed anyway and have no nutritional value.

FRED:

From tomato sauce to most frozen dinners, added sugar can be found in even the most unexpected products. Sugar is a cheap preservative, enhances taste and is highly addictive. It is therefore the perfect "weapon" for industrials to use and make their shareholders billions of dollars. A great book by Christophe Brusset ("*Vous êtes fous d'avaler ça*" / "*You are crazy to eat that*") shows that many CEOs and traders from the food industry do not, under any circumstances, feed their family their own products.

Many people rely on quick, processed foods for meals and snacks. Since these products often contain added sugar, it makes up a large proportion of their daily calorie intake. In the US, added sugars (just sugar, not total carbs) account for up to 18% of the total calorie intake of adults and up to 15% for children. It's HUGE! Dietary guidelines suggest limiting calories from added sugar to less than 10% per day, and I believe this is still way too high for our health and optimal weight.

Most scientists and nutritionists have finally accepted that sugar consumption is a major cause of obesity and many chronic diseases, such as type-2 diabetes and type-3 diabetes (aka Alzheimer's Disease). Additionally, consuming too much sugar, especially from sugar-sweetened drinks, has been linked to atherosclerosis, a disease characterized by fatty, artery-clogging deposits.

Read the study here:

https://www.ncbi.nlm.nih.gov/pmc/articles/PMC570 8308/

Another study of over 30,000 people found that those who consumed 17–21% of calories from added sugar had a 38% greater risk of dying from heart disease, compared to those consuming only 8% of calories from added sugar:

https://www.ncbi.nlm.nih.gov/pubmed/24493081

Just one 16oz. (473mL.) can of soda contains 52gr. of sugar, which equates to more than 10% of your daily calorie consumption, based on a 2,000-calorie diet. This means that one single sugary drink a day can already put you over the recommended daily limit for added sugar.

A diet high in refined carbohydrates, including grains, sugary foods and drinks, has also been associated with a higher risk of developing skin problems such as acne, eczema and psoriasis.

Eating excessive amounts of carbs and sugar also increases your risk of developing certain cancers:

- First, a diet rich in grains, sugary foods and beverages can lead to obesity, which significantly raises your risk of cancer.

- Furthermore, diets high in carbs and sugar increase inflammation in your body and directly cause insulin resistance, both of which increase cancer risk.

A study of over 430,000 people found that added sugar consumption was positively associated with an increased risk of esophageal cancer, pleural cancer and cancer of the small intestine.

Read the study here:

https://www.ncbi.nlm.nih.gov/pmc/articles/PMC349 4407/

More research on the link between sugar and disease:

https://www.medpagetoday.com/upload/2013/3/1/j ournal.pone.0057873.pdf

https://www.ncbi.nlm.nih.gov/pubmed/19211821

https://www.sciencedirect.com/science/article/abs/ pii/0306987783900956

4. Lifestyle

It is obvious that changing lifestyle only for the time of healing and returning to "pro-cancer" habits right after, would be a big mistake.

We have chosen to persevere with our protocol, in a more flexible way, of course, but keeping the main principles of regular fasting, intermittent fasting, the rawest and freshest ketogenic nutrition possible, exposure to the sun, physical exercise, breathing, stress management, etc.

This rediscovered "protocol flexibility" allows us to go to restaurants a little more often, to treat ourselves to a small dessert from time to time, but never in excess, and almost always followed by a day of fasting in order to "clean up". the organism.

PART 6: Times are changing... Evolution and oppositions

GUY:

The people vs the system... Rights vs duties

Where official medicine has already dug my grave and those of millions of cancer patients, I now intend to bring a glimmer of hope. If I have regained my health, it is no longer to enjoy it selfishly. If cancer made me live the most painful hours of my life, it also put me on a path of knowledge, experience and sharing. Today my fight continues to help develop research and share it with as many people as possible, using the tools of my YouTube channel and the scientific publications of the professors who follow me.

If my recovery is a great personal success, it is not enough because if I fought so hard, it is also to carry loud and clear the voice of the sick people for whom no real solution is provided. I made dozens of calls to several administrations which remained unanswered. I wrote to all those who could help us, have the power to change things, an audience to spread my message: a cure is possible, I have done it, I want to share it. It is time to recognize that it is possible to cure "terminal" cancer. I asked for help from the authorities: the French Ministry of Health, the National Cancer Institute, the French Cancer Foundation, the Pasteur Institute. I requested funding of up to 50,000 euros to finalize our study in a recognized independent laboratory to prove the effectiveness of our treatment. This is my life's new goal: to fight not for my own life but for that of all cancer patients around the globe. It is time to recognize the rights of patients, in particular terminal cancer patients who are only offered end-of-life palliative care. Our administrations have duties, those of proposing solutions where they do exist, by financing therapeutic trials on natural products which have proven their worth scientifically. Just because I didn't use a chemical treatment to heal myself doesn't mean that I can't be heard. Our method is in no way alternative because 100% of the pillars of my healing, which are autophagy, a 100% natural keto diet and antioxidant supplementation, come directly from the study of Nobel Prize winners in biochemistry and medicine. I don't believe in miracles; I'm not an exception but a cancer survivor who wasn't supposed to live. I tested many things; I made the decision to be a guinea pig who had everything to gain and nothing to lose. It was my most fundamental right to test these methods. It is now up to the different administrations to do something with it.

Big pharma develops treatments that cost millions of dollars each year. Current allopathic treatments have an alarming failure rate. Chemotherapy, for example, shows a failure rate of 96% after 7 years. In Europe, the market for these treatments represents $150 billion. The treatments for which I request therapeutic trials only cost a few dollars and are easily accessible, everywhere, for everyone.

Does this mean that there would not be enough profit to be made from these natural methods?

What do you think of the doctors on whom Big Pharma imposes to prescribe extremely expensive chemical treatments and menace them to revoke their licenses if they don't? I myself am in contact with renowned professors whose names I still have to keep confidential in order to protect their reputations, their careers and maybe even their lives. Millions of dollars are spent each year on research against cancer. Unfortunately, most of the studies still focus on the genetic track which is completely obsolete. At a time when epigenetics has proven that our genes react to our environment and lifestyle, it is urgent to consider the metabolic path for the future of the fight against cancer.

I put into practice powerful tools that brought me healing, both through their anti-cancer action and their health benefits. The protocol that I now wish to see developed also represents the future of integrative medicine and combines science, clinical trials and natural principles. We have everything to gain by having the different disciplines communicate with each other, because as cancer is multifactorial, so is its cure!

Both health and disease respond to a complex set of co-dependent factors that urgently need to be considered. Taking care of a sick person means first of all giving them hope.

PART 7: Q&A

Q: I'm too skinny to fast. What can I do?

A: If you're very skinny to begin with, strict fasting may be not the best thing for you. In this case, switch to a 23-1 intermittent fasting protocol, with one meal a day, made of a few raw vegetables and a large amount of good fats (avocado, nuts, sardines in olive oil, etc.) + DHA 500 supplement

Q: Should I keep taking my supplements during prolonged fasting?

A: It depends! Ideally, yes, and that's what Guy did. Fred couldn't stand them on an empty stomach and therefore stopped all supplements during his 21-day fast.

Q: How is it possible to fast for 21 days? Isn't it dangerous?

A: No, it is not dangerous if done intelligently and with common sense. If necessary, get medical attention. The human body stores energy in the form of fat, in order to cope with periods of fasting. If you are getting fatter and fatter every year, it is because you are storing without ever using these stockpiles... It is time to fast ;-)

Q: What did you eat during your prolonged water fast?

A: Water

Q: How did you stay so disciplined during all that time?

A: It's very easy when it's either that or death.

Q: Should I eat whole raw vegetables or fresh juices?

A: Again, it depends. Guy couldn't stand juices. They were giving him diarrhea, so he ate his vegetables whole. Fred couldn't stand the insoluble fiber in the vegetables, which irritated his already inflamed intestines. So, he consumed all his vegetables in the form of fresh, homemade juice.

Q: Can you tell us one more time what are the "5 essentials"?

A: #1 fasting and ketogenic diet + DHA 500
        #2 Pr. Maurice Israel's metabolic treatment (Garcinia Cambogia, Alpha Lipoic Acid, COQ10)
        #3 melatonin
        #4 matcha green tea
        #5 garlic

Q: What are the two drugs Guy mentioned that he couldn't reveal on YouTube. Drugs that apparently already exist and that would have an incredible effect in the fight against cancer?

A: Nuronefrex and Octreotide

Q: I can't sleep. Do you have any tips?

A: Sleeping can be complicated when you have cancer. We don't have anything that works 100% but some tips can help. Relaxation, meditation, deep breathing, physical activities during the day, acupuncture, chamomile herbal tea, medical marijuana...

Q: Do you still take your anti-cancer supplements even now that you are healed?

A: Yes

Q: Do you eat fruits again since you are disease-free?

A: Guy no, except berries
       Fred, yes, but only during the summer

Q: Are you both still in ketosis? Fred, what do you think of keto/carb-cycle? Can we imagine post cancer a ketogenic diet with carbohydrate days (very moderate: like green vegetables / low-fat proteins and a little potato and fruit)?

A: Fred: Absolutely. Personally, I do eat fruits again (mainly in the summer) about 3 days a week. Back on a ketogenic diet the other days. I never do nonfat proteins though. I always eat meat with the highest possible saturated fat ratio (ribeye steak, lamb, salmon, etc.).

Q: Should I try to gain weight before a fast?

A: Why not, but be careful not to feed the tumor with a diet that is too rich in growth factor foods. Above all, do not "stuff yourself" before a fast.

Q: For Fred: After remission, still a fan of the 80/20? Or rather 95/05 for the rest of your life? Cheese for example, after cancer, it is rather *never* or *occasionally* (raw milk cheese of course)

A: Closer to 90/10 for the moment indeed because my intestines are still sensitive. I eat cheese occasionally (once a week maximum and always from raw milk and 100% grass-fed).

Q: Can fasting be used against all forms of cancer?

A: We believe so, but this is just a personal opinion. Being neither doctors nor biologists, we cannot answer with certainty. Just sharing our experience and research.

Q: Apparently, Glutamine might be an alternative fuel for cancer when one is not eating any sugar... Is bone broth really recommended then? What about organ meat?

A: Fred: I ate a lot (and still do) of red meat, organs (beef liver) and home-made bone broth. All organic, pasture-raised and grass-fed. BUT, I always have a big cup of Matcha green tea with those, to control glutamine levels and I also supplemented with DHA

Q: How does Fred look so young for a 50-year-old guy? (don't laugh, we did get this question dozens of times)

A: Probably because I never drank alcohol in my life, never smoked, never had soda or "junk-food", played sports all my life, and practiced intermittent fasting for almost 20 years). Also, I laugh a lot. Laughter and joy are great antioxidants.

PART 8: Fred's keto recipes

If for any reason you cannot buy organic, be aware of the EWG's Dirty Dozen, the twelve worst pesticide-heavy foods to eat:

1. *Strawberries*
2. *Spinach*
3. *Kale*
4. *Nectarines*
5. *Apples*
6. *Grapes*
7. *Peaches*
8. *Cherries*
9. *Pears*
10. *Tomatoes*
11. *Celery*
12. *Potatoes*

The following recipes are for four persons, but of course, if it seems too much or too little for you and your family, adapt the portions to your appetite. Stop eating when you are full, but make sure you have enough daily calories, fats and proteins. A lot of people, when starting a Ketogenic diet do not eat enough because the fat fills them up more than the carbs.

I. French influence

- Slow cooked pork or lamb shoulder "à la cuillère"

Ingredients:
1 bone-in shoulder of pork or lamb
2 tbsp. of organic cold-pressed olive oil
3 tbsp. of organic 100% grass-fed butter
6 cups of bone broth
Pink Himalayan salt
Pepper
Garlic powder
Onion powder

Preparation and cooking:
Remove meat from fridge 1h. before cooking.

20min. before cooking brush with olive oil then season with salt, pepper, garlic and onion powder on both sides.

In a sauté pan, brown the meat in butter or ghee on all sides at high temperature.

Then lower the temperature to the minimum, cover the meat with bone broth, cover and cook for 3h. (lamb) or 4h. (pork). Half way through, flip the meat to the other side. Baste the meat with its bone broth every 30min. to prevent it from drying out.

Serve with any vegetable you want.

Note about butter: High quality butter is golden-yellow. If it's white or light in color, it's low quality, processed and grain-fed.

- **"Poulet à la crème" heavy-cream chicken with mushrooms**

Ingredients:
8 boneless chicken thighs with skin
1 tbsp. of organic 100% grass-fed ghee
1 cup of organic grass-fed heavy cream
Pink Himalayan salt
Pepper
Garlic powder
Onion powder
3 cups of fresh organic mushrooms, minced

Preparation and cooking:
Remove meat from fridge 30min. before cooking.

20min. before cooking, brush with olive oil, then season with salt, pepper, garlic and onion powder on both sides.

In a sauté pan, brown the meat in butter or ghee on all sides at high temperature.

Then lower the temperature to the minimum, cover the meat with the heavy cream, add the minced mushrooms, cover and cook for 20min.

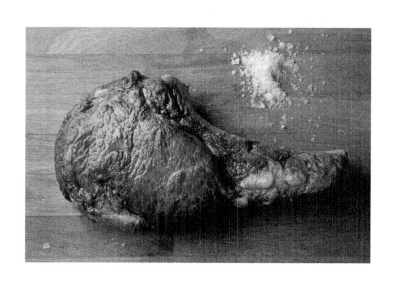

- **"Cote de bœuf 2 cuissons" Bone-in Ribeye cooked twice**

Ingredients:
1 extra thick grass-fed bone-in Ribeye (2.5 inches thick or more)
2 tbsp. of organic 100% grass-fed butter or ghee
2 tbsp. of organic cold-pressed olive oil
Pink Himalayan salt
Pepper
Garlic powder
Onion powder
Herbs of your choice (thyme, oregano...)

Preparation and cooking:
Remove meat from fridge 1h. before cooking.

Brush with olive oil, then season with salt, pepper, garlic and onion powder on both sides.

In a sauté pan, brown the meat in butter or ghee on all sides at high temperature.

Pre-heat your oven to 400°F (200°C).

Put the meat in an oven safe baking dish (or even better, a cast-iron pan if you have one). Cook for about 6min. per pound (see chart bellow).

VERY IMPORTANT: Red meat needs to "rest" for about 8min. before serving. It's going to be much juicer and more tender. Add butter and "fleur de sel de Guérande" ET VOILA!

SIRLOIN STRIP STEAKS, RIBEYE STEAKS & PORTERHOUSE STEAKS

Thickness	Rare 110° To 120° F	Medium Rare 120° To 130° F	Medium 130° To 140° F
1"	4 minutes EACH SIDE	5 minutes EACH SIDE	6 minutes EACH SIDE
1.25"	4.5 minutes EACH SIDE	5.5 minutes EACH SIDE	6.5 minutes EACH SIDE
1.5"	5 minutes EACH SIDE	6 minutes EACH SIDE	7 minutes EACH SIDE
1.75"	5.5 minutes EACH SIDE	6.5 minutes EACH SIDE	7.5 minutes EACH SIDE
2"	6 minutes EACH SIDE	7 minutes EACH SIDE	8 minutes EACH SIDE

- **"Pot-au-feu" home-made bone broth with bone marrow, short ribs and winter vegetables** (for 1 week of bone broth for 4 people)

Ingredients:
For the broth:
2 lbs. of grass-fed beef marrowbones
2 lbs. of grass-fed beef short ribs
1 lbs. of grass-fed oxtail
Pink Himalayan salt
Pepper
Garlic and onion powder
1 tbsp. of organic raw apple cider vinegar
1 gallon of water

Vegetables:
Turnips
Zucchini
Celery
Onions
Garlic

Preparation and cooking:
Put all the bone broth ingredients in a Crockpot or slow cooker. Cover with water (to 3 inches above food line) and slow cook for 24h.

Add all the veggies and continue to cook for another 45min.

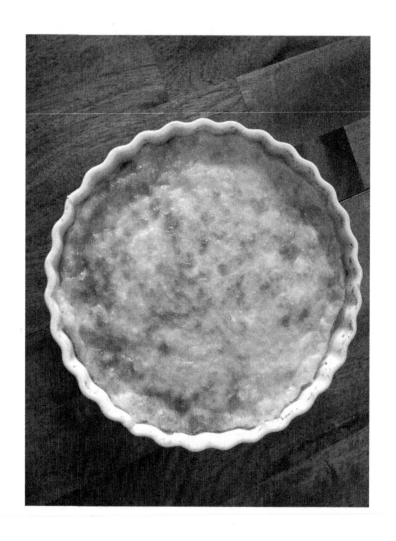

- **Crustless French quiche**

Ingredients:
5 organic eggs
250 ml. of organic heavy cream
1/2 lbs. of sugar-free bacon
1 cup of organic grass-fed grated Swiss cheese (you could use cheddar but remember that it's one of the most processed cheese out there)
Pink Himalayan salt
Pepper

Preparation and cooking:
Cut and pre-cook the bacon in a pan and set aside.

Mix the eggs with the cream in a food processor.

Mix all ingredients together (reserving ¼ cup of cheese) and put everything in a deep-dish pie pan, cover with the reserved cheese.

Cook at 300°F (150°C) for 30-40min. until golden-brown.

Let the quiche rest for 20min. Enjoy!

- **Crustless warm camembert pie**

<u>Ingredients</u>:
5 organic eggs
250 ml. of organic heavy cream
1 French raw-milk Camembert
1 cup of organic grass-fed grated Swiss cheese (you could use cheddar but remember that it's one of the most processed cheese out there)
Pink Himalayan salt
Pepper

<u>Preparation and cooking</u>:
Mix eggs, cream and ¾ cup Swiss cheese in a food processor.

Pour egg mixture in a deep-dish pie pan, put the whole Camembert in the center and cover with a the reserved ¼ cup Swiss cheese.

Cook at 300°F (150°C) for 30-40min. until golden-brown.

Let the Camembert pie rest for 20min. Enjoy!

- **"Cuisses de canard confit" duck confit**

<u>Ingredients</u>:
4 duck legs with bone and skin
1 clove of organic garlic
Pink Himalayan salt
Pepper
3 tbsp. of organic duck fat

<u>Preparation and cooking</u>:
Remove meat from fridge 1h. before cooking.

Season with salt and pepper on both sides.

In a sauté pan, brown the meat in duck fat on both sides at high temperature until skin is crispy (about 10min.).

Lower the temperature, add the garlic, cover the pan and cook for another 30min.

Serve with garlic cauliflower mash (aka "mashed ketatoes") instead of high-carb mashed potatoes.

II. Asian influence

- **Thai lemongrass chicken thighs with cauliflower rice**

Ingredients:
Organic free-range boneless chicken thighs with skin
3 tbsp. of organic coconut oil
1 clove of organic garlic
Sugar-free Thai red curry paste
2 chopped stalks of lemongrass
Fresh Cilantro
3 kaffir lime leaves

Preparation and cooking:
Marinate the chicken with the red curry paste, the chopped lemongrass, chopped Cilantro and the chopped kaffir lime leaves in the fridge overnight.

Get the marinated chicken out of the fridge 20min. before cooking it.

In a sauté pan, brown the thighs in coconut oil on skin side at high temperature until skin is crispy.

Then lower the temperature, flip the thighs, add the garlic and cook the other side for another 2-3min. Serve with cauliflower rice and sautéed Bok Choy.

- **"Fong Kai" Hakka-style red chicken**

Ingredients:
Organic free-range boneless chicken thighs with skin
3 tbsp. of organic coconut oil
1 clove of organic garlic
Sugar-free red chili pepper sauce
¼ cup of gluten-free organic Tamari or soy sauce
Pink Himalayan salt
1 tsp. of Chinese 5-spice powder
½ gallon of homemade bone broth

Preparation and cooking:
Remove meat from fridge 30min. before cooking.

In a large stockpot, brown the thighs in coconut oil on both sides at high temperature until skin is crispy.

Lower the temperature, add the garlic, chili sauce, salt, Chinese 5-spice and soy sauce, cover everything with bone broth.

Cover the pan and cook for another 1h.

Serve the red chicken in a bowl with the cooking liquid, and sides of cauliflower rice and sautéed Bok Choy.

- **Thai coconut green curry with duck**

Ingredients:
4 free-range duck breasts with skin
1 tbsp. of organic coconut oil
Sugar-free Thai green curry paste
2 cups of organic coconut cream
2 chopped kaffir lime leaves
Pink Himalayan salt
16 baby Thai eggplants (cut in half)

Preparation and cooking:
Get the duck out of the fridge 30min. before cooking it.

In a sauté pan, brown the thighs in coconut oil on both sides at high temperature, until skin is crispy.

Transfer duck to a large saucepan and add remaining ingredients. Cook over low heat for 20min. until eggplants are fully cooked (they should be soft)

- **Chinese-style beef**

Ingredients:
4 16-oz organic grass-fed Ribeyes
3 tbsp. of organic coconut oil
1 clove of organic garlic
2 tbsp. of organic gluten-free Tamari or Soy sauce
Pink Himalayan salt
5-spice powder
Onion powder

Preparation and cooking:
Marinate the ribeyes with the soy sauce, 5-spice and onion powder, salt and garlic in the fridge for at least 3h (overnight is even better).

Remove marinated beef from fridge 1h. before cooking.

In a sauté pan or a wok, cook the Ribeyes in coconut oil on both sides at high temperature. Cook to your liking. I recommend medium-rare.

Let the meat rest for 6min. and cut into thick slices.

Serve with cauliflower rice and any vegetables you desire.

- Chinese-style garlic shrimp with fried rice

Ingredients:
2 lbs. of fresh shrimp
2 tbsp. of organic coconut oil
1 clove of organic garlic
4 tbsp. of organic gluten-free soy sauce
Pink Himalayan salt
1 tbsp. of Chinese cooking wine Shao Xing
Cauliflower rice
4 bunches of broccolini
Chives

Preparation and cooking:
Marinate the shrimp with the salt, half of the soy sauce and garlic in the fridge for at least 2h.

Remove the marinated shrimp from the fridge 10min. before cooking.

In a sauté pan or a wok, cook the shrimp in coconut oil with the broccolini, and the wine until caramelized and put aside.

Then, on medium heat, cook the cauliflower rice in coconut oil with the remaining soy sauce until dry. Add the shrimp, veggies and chives.

Cook for another 2min. and enjoy.

- **Vietnamese low-carb Pho soup**

Ingredients:
Homemade bone broth
4 8-oz. grass-fed beef filet
1 lbs. of grass-fed beef brisket
4 packages of organic shirataki "miracle noodles"
1 clove of organic garlic, minced
2 onions, sliced
4 spring onion butts
3 star-anise
2 cloves
1/3 cup of organic gluten-free soy sauce
Pink Himalayan salt
Fresh cilantro
Fresh basil
2 handfuls of soybean sprouts

Preparation and cooking:
Cut the filet into thin slices and marinate with the garlic, 1 onion, soy sauce and salt in the fridge for at least 1h.

Remove the marinated beef from the fridge 1h. before putting it in the soup.

Rinse the shirataki noodle very carefully, cook them in salted boiling water and dry them in a pan as indicated in the directions. Set aside.

Cook the brisket in the bone broth together with star anise, cloves and spring onion butts. When brisket is cooked, remove the ingredients.

Put the noodles in 4 separate large bowls. Put raw beef and cooked brisket on top and pour in the very hot broth. Add remaining onion, basil, cilantro and soybean sprouts. Enjoy!

- **Filipino chicken Adobo**

Ingredients:
4 packages of organic shirataki "miracle rice"
8 organic chicken thighs
1 cup of apple cider vinegar
1 cup of organic gluten-free soy sauce
½ cup of garlic, minced
3 tbsp. of organic coconut oil
1 organic onion, sliced
2 tbsp. of black pepper
Himalayan pink salt
4 bay leaves
2 cups of bone broth

Preparation and cooking:
Prepare miracle rice as indicated on package.

Marinade chicken with soy sauce, vinegar, black pepper and garlic for at least 1h.

In a large pan, brown chicken in coconut oil (2 tbsp.), then remove and set aside.

In the same pan, add the remaining coconut oil and sauté onions with salt until soft then stir-fry everything for 1min.

Add the browned chicken, marinade sauce, bay leaves, bone broth and simmer covered until the chicken is tender.

Remove chicken and place on top of rice. Simmer the sauce until thickened then pour onto the chicken and rice.

Optional: You can add spring onions to garnish.

- "Kim Chu Niou" Cantonese golden pork

Ingredients:
2.5 lbs. of pork belly, with skin
1.5 tbsp. Chinese cooking wine Shao Xing
1 tsp. Chinese 5-spice powder
1 tsp. white pepper (sub black pepper)
½ tsp. pink Himalayan salt
1 tbsp. white vinegar
5 oz. (140 gr.) of grey rock salt

Preparation and cooking:
Use an ice pick, sharp metal skewer or another tool to prick tons and tons of holes in the skin. Avoid piercing into the fat as best as you can, and really ensure you do not pierce the flesh.

Turn the pork belly upside down. Rub the flesh (not the skin) with Chinese cooking wine, dribbling it on gradually. Sprinkle over the 5-spice powder, pink salt and pepper. Rub all over flesh, including sides (again, not on skin).

Turn skin side up and place in a container. Dab skin dry with paper towels. Refrigerate uncovered for 12-24h.

Preheat oven to 350°F (180°C)

Remove pork from fridge. Place onto a large sheet

of foil. Fold up sides of foil around the pork to enclose it snugly with a 2/5" (1.5 cm.) rim above the pork skin (to hold the rock salt in).

Transfer pork to baking tray. Dab skin with paper towels and brush skin with vinegar.

Spread rock salt on the skin (the foil edges will stop it from falling down the sides).

Roast for 50-60min.

Then remove pork from oven and transfer onto work surface.

Switch to grill/broiler on medium high. Move shelf so it is about 10" (25cm.) from the heat source.

Fold down foil and scrape all the salt off the top and sides. Return pork to baking tray and place under grill/broiler for 20min., rotating tray once, until skin is golden, crispy and puffed.

III. International influence

- **Organic bunless cheeseburger**

Ingredients:
3lbs. of organic grass-fed ground beef (preferably 75% lean 25% fat)
1 tbsp. of organic ghee
Pink Himalayan salt
Pepper
Garlic powder
Onion powder
8 slices of organic raw-milk Swiss cheese
8 large lettuce wraps
1 organic tomato
Organic guacamole (homemade if possible)

Preparation and cooking:
Prepare your patties with ground beef, salt, onion and garlic powder (I usually count 0.75lbs. per person but not everyone eats as much as I do...)

Grill the burger on an outdoor grill - or in a frying pan with ghee - on one side. Flip them and immediately add the cheese so it has time to melt.

Prepare your lettuce wraps with the guacamole and slices of tomatoes. Put the patties with melted cheese on top. Enjoy!

- **Grilled Ribeye, mashed "ketatoes" and asparagus**

Ingredients:
4 thick grass-fed Ribeye (2 inches thick)
2 tbsp. of organic cold-pressed olive oil
Pink Himalayan salt
Guérande fleur de sel
Pepper
Garlic powder
Onion powder
Asparagus

For the mashed "ketatoes":
2 heads of organic cauliflower, cut into florets
2 tbsp. of 100% grass-fed butter
1 cup of 100% grass-fed heavy cream
½ cup of organic cream cheese
Enough bone broth to cook the cauliflower
2 garlic cloves, minced
Pink Himalayan salt
Pepper

Preparation and cooking:
Remove meat from the fridge 1h. before cooking.

20min. before cooking, brush the ribeyes and the asparagus with olive oil and season with salt, pepper, garlic and onion powder.

Pre-heat your BBQ grill to 400°F (200°C).

Cook the Ribeyes to your liking (using the chart below).

3min. before meat is done put the asparagus on the grill.

Let the meat rest for 8min. before serving.

For the garlic mashed "ketatoes":

Put the cauliflower, salt and broth in a large pot. Cover and cook until the cauliflower is tender.

Drain the liquid, and squeeze excess from the cauliflower by placing it between 2 paper towels. Get as much as liquid out as possible for a better "mashed potato" effect.

In a food processor, combine the cooked cauliflower with all the cream, butter, cream cheese, garlic, salt and pepper. Purée until smooth.

Better prepare the mashed "ketatoes" before cooking the meat and reheat before eating.

SIRLOIN STRIP STEAKS, RIBEYE STEAKS & PORTERHOUSE STEAKS

Thickness	Rare 110° To 120° F	Medium Rare 120° To 130° F	Medium 130° To 140° F
1"	4 minutes EACH SIDE	5 minutes EACH SIDE	6 minutes EACH SIDE
1.25"	4.5 minutes EACH SIDE	5.5 minutes EACH SIDE	6.5 minutes EACH SIDE
1.5"	5 minutes EACH SIDE	6 minutes EACH SIDE	7 minutes EACH SIDE
1.75"	5.5 minutes EACH SIDE	6.5 minutes EACH SIDE	7.5 minutes EACH SIDE
2"	6 minutes EACH SIDE	7 minutes EACH SIDE	8 minutes EACH SIDE

VERY IMPORTANT: Red meat needs to "rest" 6-8min. before serving. It's going to be much juicer and more tender. Add a butter and "fleur de sel" and enjoy!

- **Unilaterally cooked salmon**

Ingredients:
4 thick wild caught salmon fillets with skin
2 tbsp. of organic cold-pressed olive or avocado oil
Pink Himalayan salt
Pepper
1 lemon

Preparation and cooking:
Remove salmon from the fridge 15min. before cooking. Season with salt and pepper.

In a sauté pan on medium heat, cook the salmon in oil on skin side only. DO NOT FLIP IT. When you can see from the sides that the fillet is cooked halfway through, the salmon is ready.

Serve on 4 plates. Squeeze fresh lemon juice on top. Side with any vegetable you like.

Enjoy your meal.

- **Keto cobb salad**

Ingredients:
8 cups of organic lettuce or mixed green salad
4 organic eggs
2 cups of cherry tomatoes
1/2 lbs. of sugar-free bacon
1 cup of organic Roquefort (French sheep-milk blue cheese)
4 organic avocados
Pink Himalayan salt
Pepper
Organic cold-pressed olive oil
Organic apple cider vinegar

Preparation and cooking:
Soft boil the eggs and let them cool down.

Cut and pre-cook the bacon in a pan.

Cut/slice all ingredients.

Put everything in a large bowl, cover with a little extra cheese.

Prepare your vinaigrette with the oil, vinegar, salt and pepper – Ratio is 2tbsp. of oil for 1tbsp. of vinegar.

- **Grass-fed cheese Keto wrap**

Ingredients:
2 cups of organic raw-milk shredded Swiss cheese (real Swiss or gruyere should always be from grass-fed milk)
2 cups of organic shredded mozzarella
Pink Himalayan salt
Pepper

Preparation and cooking:
Mix all ingredients together.

Form the mixture in a pancake-like shape on a cooking sheet.

Bake in the oven at 350°F (150°C) until golden-brown.

Let the cheese wraps cool down for 2min.

Use them like regular wrap and put anything you'd like in them... Chicken, ham, guacamole, tomatoes, lettuce, bell peppers, onions...

- **Keto pizza**

<u>Ingredients</u> (for an 8-slice pie):
Dough:
2.5 cups of organic shredded mozzarella
1 cup of almond flour
¼ cup of coconut flour
2 organic eggs
½ tsp. organic apple cider vinegar
Pink Himalayan salt

Toppings:
Sugar-free organic tomato sauce
2 cups of fresh mozzarella, sliced
(see homemade mozzarella recipe below)
+ Anything you like. I usually simply put cheese, garlic and mushrooms on my pizza.

<u>Preparation and cooking</u>:
Melt the mozzarella cheese in a double boiler or in the microwave (I'm not a fan of microwave but it's the easiest and fastest).

Add the eggs and the vinegar to the melted cheese and mix in a food processor. Keep mixing and add the dry ingredients. Finish it by hand so all the ingredients are well combined together.

On a cooking sheet and with a rolling pin, add the coconut flour and roll out the dough as thin as you can without breaking it (crust will feel weird if too thick).

Precook crust in the oven at 450°F (230°C) for 7min. on each side (yes, you have to flip the crust and cook it on both sides), until it starts to get crispy.

Remove crust from oven and add the tomato base first, and all the toppings finishing with the cheese.

Bake the whole pie at 450°F (230°C) for another 6-8min. until cheese has melted.

And please I'm begging you: no tabasco or pineapple on pizza!

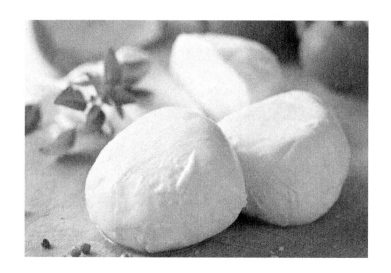

- **Make your own mozzarella** (it's super easy)

Ingredients:
½ gallon of organic whole raw milk
½ cup of organic white vinegar
½ handful of pink Himalayan salt
A medium size bowl with ice-cold water (for the very last part of the recipe)

Preparation and cooking:
Pour milk in a large saucepan and heat until 120°F (50°C).

Turn off the heat and add the vinegar. Cover immediately to trap the steam.

Let it sit for 4min. to let the curd form at the surface. Scoop the curd out with a fine mesh strainer but keep the whey-water in the pot.

Start turning the cheese with a spoon or a spatula, gently pressing against the strainer. As you turn and get the excess water out of the curd, you will see your cheese forming.

Turn the heat back up underneath the pot to warm up the whey-water and add the salt (low heat).

Rest the cheese in the whey-water (to flavor it with the salt in the water). Remove cheese again with strainer and turn it again to get the stretchiness. Repeat the operation one more time.

Work the cheese by hand to form a nice soft ball and put the ball in ice-cold water for 5min.

Put cheese in paper towel to dry it just a little and it's ready. Fresh homemade mozzarella.

Here is the video from which I learned to make my own mozzarella, from Sweet Adjeley's Youtube Channel:

https://www.youtube.com/watch?v=QXotHLGyZEQ&t=178s

- Keto enchiladas

Ingredients:
1lbs. of all-natural sliced chicken breast (from the deli counter preferably)
1lbs. of organic 100% grass-fed ground beef
1 cup of organic raw-milk shredded Swiss cheese
1 cup of organic shredded mozzarella
2 tbsp. of organic cold-pressed avocado oil
Pink Himalayan salt
Pepper
Sugar-free organic tomato sauce or salsa
½ tbsp. chopped onion
½ tbsp. chopped fresh cilantro.
1 jalapeño pepper, seeded and chopped

Preparation and cooking:
Remove the meat from the fridge 1h. before cooking.

In a sauté pan, brown your ground meat in avocado oil at medium temperature.

Then mix the meat with the tomato sauce, the onions, the cilantro, the jalapeño, salt, pepper and the mozzarella cheese (not the Swiss yet).

Pre-heat your oven to 400°F (204°C).

Use the slices of chicken breast just as if they were tortillas. Fill them up with the mixture and roll them up.

Put the rolled enchiladas in an oven safe baking dish, add a little more tomato sauce, top with some Swiss cheese, and bake for 10min.

- African chicken stew with coconut cauliflower rice

<u>Ingredients</u>:
4 organic free-range chicken leg quarters with skin
4 ripe organic tomatoes
½ cup + 1 tbsp. of organic coconut cream
3 tbsp. of organic coconut oil
1 tsp. of curry powder
1 tsp. of paprika
1 tsp. of onion powder
1 large onion
1 clove of garlic, minced
1 tbsp. of organic peanut butter
1 handful of scallions, chopped
Pink Himalayan salt
Pepper
Thyme
2 cups of homemade bone broth
½ cup of shredded coconut (dry)
Cauliflower rice

<u>Preparation and cooking</u>:
Remove chicken from the fridge 20min. before cooking. With a knife, separate thighs and drumsticks

In a large stockpot, brown the thighs in coconut oil (2 tbsp.) on both sides at high temperature until skin is crispy. Set aside.

Using the same pot (without washing it) put the tomatoes, onion, minced garlic, curry powder, paprika and thyme and cook them for 10min.

Add the bone broth, the peanut butter and ½ cup coconut cream. Mix everything well and add the chicken.

Cover and cook everything at low temperature for 30min.

For the coconut cauliflower rice:
Sauté the rice in coconut oil (1 tbsp.) with shredded coconut and 1 tbsp. of coconut cream. Salt to your liking.

Put the rice and stew in one or two separate bowls (up to you), add the scallions on top of the chicken stew. Enjoy!

- Keto chicken-lamb Couscous

Ingredients (for 6 to 8 people):
4 organic chicken legs with skin
1 lamb shoulder confit (see recipe above)
Organic olive oil
Organic butter
Pink Himalayan salt
Pepper
Saffron
Coriander powder
1 liter of bone broth
4 ripe organic tomatoes
3 zucchini
8 turnips
1 onion
1 clove of garlic
3 large cauliflowers

Preparation and cooking:
Prepare the shoulder of lamb as indicated in the recipe.

Take the chicken out of the refrigerator 20min. before cooking. Cut the thighs in half and season with salt and pepper.

In a frying pan, brown the chicken legs over high heat in olive oil until the skin is golden brown. Set aside.

Wash and peel your vegetables and put them in a large pot with the bone broth, salt, pepper, saffron and coriander powder.

Cover and cook on low heat for 30 to 40 minutes.

For cauliflower couscous:
Put the <u>raw</u> cauliflower in a blender until the size is about the size of a grain of couscous, then cook it in a large frying pan with both olive oil and butter.

Before serving, heat lamb and chicken with a little bone broth.

IV. Fresh vegetable juices

Here is an interesting article on juicing and oncology:

https://www.oncologynutrition.org/erfc/healthy-nutrition-now/foods/should-i-be-juicing

Here are several examples of juices that I make in order to regain full health (remember that it is essential to use seasonal and organic fruits and vegetables). I changed a few recipes from my first book. During the four months of fighting, there were no fruits or root vegetables in my juices. I added carrots, beets and berries only after the tumor was gone.

These "recipes" are for one person.

Juice #1:

¼ lbs. of kale
1 handfull of blueberries
1 inch of fresh turmeric (curcumin)

Juice #2:

¼ lbs. of parsley
3 purple carrots

1 inch of fresh turmeric (curcumin)
½ a lemon

Juice #3:

¼ lbs. of baby spinach
1 handful of blueberries
1 stalk of celery
1 inch of fresh turmeric (curcumin)

Juice #4:

¼ lbs. of collards
1 tsp of apple cider vinegar
1 lemon
1 inch of fresh turmeric (curcumin)

Juice #5:

¼ lbs. of pak choy
3 stalks of celery
1 handful of raspberries
1 inch of fresh turmeric (curcumin)

Juice #6:

3 multi-color carrots

1 lemon
1 inch of fresh turmeric (curcumin)

Juice #7:

¼ lbs. of baby spinach
1 lemon
1 red cabbage
1 inch of fresh turmeric (curcumin)

Juice #8:

¼ lbs. of kale
3 carrots
5 strawberries
1 inch of fresh turmeric (curcumin)

Juice #9 (my favorite, for special days):

6 carrots
1 beetroot
1 handful of spinach
1 blood orange
1 inch of fresh turmeric (curcumin)

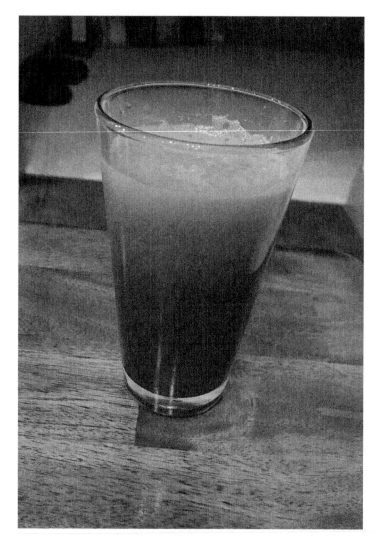

Juice #9

A few words from our spouses

From Lila (Fred's wife)

The day Fred was diagnosed with cancer, my whole world collapsed. We always believed that this couldn't happen to us because of our healthy lifestyle! I remember I was at home in the US with only my puppy, while Fred was in France for medical exams - for what we thought was only an intestinal inflammation. He called me to tell me that the doctors said it was cancer, and it was already stage 3. I broke in tears.

The doctors said that looking at his family's cancer history and the advance stage of his cancer, he would probably be dead already if not for his healthy lifestyle and ketogenic diet. When something like that happens in your life, it puts everything else in perspectives. Cancer becomes your whole world. Since I've known him (we've been married for 18 years), Fred was always so strong and so brave... He fought so many battles in his life, but I knew that this one would be the hardest of them all.

We can't realize how difficult it is until you are in the middle of it. I saw him in so much pain; I still don't know how he did it. But I knew he would fight for his life; for me, for his family, for his students, no matter how hard.

Now, less than 4 months after being diagnosed, Fred is completely cured! I believe his 'experience' is unique because he used many different holistic tools to reach this goal and he faithfully believed that his immune system and his "warrior" mental strength could heal him more surely that any chemical and toxic treatment. I encouraged him to share his journey by writing a book, this book, as I truly believe it can help a lot of people.

Living with Fred in our house in South Carolina, and having been a direct witness of how well and fast he beat this cancer, using the traditional knowledge of fasting, nutrition, Tai Chi, meditation, etc., and refusing the heavy long-term chemotherapy, radiation and surgery oncologists told him he had to do to survive, I can say that I have never been so proud of him. He showed me, and everyone we know, what true courage is.

I am so proud of him to have fought this ultimate battle so bravely and fearlessly.

From Dominique (Guy's wife)

The day of Guy's cancer diagnosis was the worst day of my life. I couldn't believe the prognosis that he was going to disappear within three months.

Personally, I couldn't accept that he was not going to leave me. Very quickly, Guy took control of his destiny, thinking "it is impossible that there is nothing to do". He took this impossible fight head-on to finally discover new possibilities and study with the greatest professors and Nobel Prize winners around the world.

It was this research and the understanding of what cancer really was that allowed him to come out of it and live where conventional medicine had condemned him.

I discovered (or rather rediscovered) my husband and the fighter he was, and I am so proud of him.

Four years later, when we were predicted of his imminent death, we live normally again while being very attentive to his lifestyle and continuing to follow this protocol, which gave him his health back.

Guy has completely changed. The important things for him today is his family, his friends and helping cancer patients to survive; to heal. This is the challenge of his new life; life that he almost lost, four years ago already.

His subscribers nicknamed him "the Samurai", and Yes! This is exactly what he is, a true Samurai who never gave up until his final victory.

Conclusion

As you can see Fred and Guy's approaches for a cure (and not simple remission) of cancer are extremely close. If the cancer still finds its way, so does the cure.

Our salvation, we owe it to our research, our reading, and our refusal of the official medical prognosis. We researched and finally understood what cancer was, and did not allow ourselves to be influenced by the all-mighty modern oncology and its limitations. We were the architects of our decisions and our healings.

Life is self-healing! This is the principle of homeostasis, which says that any living organism left to rest in its natural environment systematically returns to a state of equilibrium.

The body is intelligent and tells us what to do, you just have to know how to listen!

A last word from Guy for his new friend Fred:

Thank you, Fred, for joining me in our fight, not for our glory but for the good of all Cancer patients.

We will continue together to help and inform people of all the discoveries that our teams make here:

Guy's YouTube Channel
YouTube.com/c/SurviveFromCancer

Fred's YouTube Channel
https://www.youtube.com/c/FredEvrardAcademy

1st **Afterword** by Doctor Jean-Marie Dessaint

INDISPENSABLE, INCONTOURNABLE, INNOVANT!

This book can save your life and the lives of those you love!

The book you are holding in your hands is certainly the most important you have ever had the opportunity to read. The story of Guy and Fred's recovery could be described as miraculous, but there is nothing miraculous about it: it is the result of a fierce desire for recovery and hard work every day and every moment that allowed them to thwart the gloomy prognosis that all these doctors had given them, both in France and in the USA, by giving Guy only a few months of life expectancy and at most two years with palliative care, and to Fred a one in two chance of getting out of it.

Their protocols and testimonials are carefully followed and supported by great French and American professors: professor and former research director at the CNRS Maurice Israel, professor Thomas Seyfried and professor Eric Berg among others, as well as naturopaths experienced in cancer treatments (Patrick Louis) who study their cases and provide them with valuable advice and assistance.

Guy is completely healed and in great shape. You can check it out by following his videos; he looks resplendent for a cancer patient at the end of life. All his examinations have returned to normal (CT scan, PET scan, bone scan, ultrasound, blood tests... and his PSA is undetectable, less than 0.1). His prostate has regained a normal volume and appearance. Not only did he recover from terminal prostate cancer with metastases, but over the course of his trials he also recovered from type 2 diabetes, Parkinson's disease, psoriasis, hypertension blood pressure, cholesterol and obesity.

Fred cured himself in just four months and returned to impressive martial and athletic performances!

But Guy and Fred are not doing this for themselves, they want to share all their discoveries with the greatest number of cancer patients, but also many other diseases. This is the subject of this very didactic and very clear book which hides nothing. He explains everything to you in a concise way. Its objective is to save the 200,000 cancer deaths each year in France and the other 650,000 in the United States, almost 10 million worldwide. But beware Guy constantly repeats that he should not be copied, he is not a doctor. If you want to apply these methods, it is absolutely necessary to be followed by a doctor and above all not to stop your treatments without the advice of your oncologist or general practitioner.

With our entire team, we are for integrative medicine, that is to say medicine that harmoniously combines official so-called "allopathic" medicine with dietetics, naturopathy, psychology, physical exercise, and everything that allows healing. by associating all the positive forces.

I hope you enjoyed this book.

-Dr. Jean-Marie Dessaint, *graduated from the Faculty of Medicine of Lille (France) and a member of the Council of the Order of Physicians of Isère (France).*

2nd **Afterword** by Doctor Charles Gibert

I dreamed about it... they did it!!!

I will not repeat here what Dr. Jean Marie Dessaint has just described so well. Like him, I remain a scientist who observes facts and seeks explanations. And here, concerning these so-called miraculous healings, I would be of very bad faith if I did not ask myself questions that challenge conventional medicine thinking. Fred's and Guy's stories, I had lived them with some of my patients before. My experience with cancer had long suggested to me that something fundamental eluded official beliefs and protocols. My holistic conception of health had long suggested to me that chance and genetics did not answer all my questions. One day, a scientist friend of mine offered me her book, written in collaboration with other researchers. It was about the mechanics of cancer, epigenetics, and a realistic, rather cruel assessment of official protocols. By reading this work, I measured what Fred and Guy clearly named "the gap between scientific research and official medicine". One keeps asking questions, exploring paradigms, differences, when the other just applies protocols, hoping for the best.

However, and this is a crucial point, a patient is an individual and must be treated as such. I have met thousands of them in my fifty years of career. It is obvious that they do not all experience disease in the same way. Some will resign themselves to a prognosis, others will not accept it. Fred, Guy and so many others, to whom the protocols, the accepted beliefs, the authorities had predicted the worst, took a different path. And here they are, in a place where conventional knowledge did not expect them... alive and well.

Their adventure raises interesting and... disturbing questions. They could have resumed a normal life, enjoying their success, quietly. But they have decided to share with the world what their journey contains of lessons and hope.

Bibliography

- My battle against cancer impossible, *Guy Tenenbaum*

- How my immune system beat cancer, *Fred Evrard*

- Eat fat to lose, *Fred Evrard*

- Cancer as a metabolic disease, *Dr. Thomas N. Seyfried*

- Keto for Cancer: Ketogenic Metabolic Therapy as a Targeted Nutritional Strategy, *Miriam Kalamian, EdM, MS, CNS*

-The metabolic approach to cancer, *Dr. Nasha Winters*

- Fat for Fuel, *Dr. Joseph Mercola*

- Guérir enfin du cancer: Oser dire quand et comment, *Pr. Henry Joyeux*

- Keto answers, *Anthony Gustin, MD and Chris Irvin*

- Lies my doctor told me, *Dr. Ken Berry*

- The Art and Science of Low Carbohydrate Living, *Dr. Stephen Phinney and Dr. Jeff Volek*
- Comment le blé moderne nous intoxique, *Dr. William Davis*

More resources for further research

The "SCOT" study:
https://jscholaronline.com/articles/JOCR/Inhibition-of-Scot-and-Ketolysis-Decreases.pdf

Guy's YouTube channel:
https://www.youtube.com/c/SurviveFromCancer

Fred's YouTube channel:
https://www.youtube.com/channel/UCnJF5tsWLdZ7mZnjM5rOGrQ

Dr. Eric Berg's YouTube channel:
https://www.youtube.com/c/DrEricBergDC

Dr. Thomas N. Seyfried - Cancer as a Metabolic Disease:
https://www.amazon.com/Cancer-Metabolic-Disease-Management-Prevention/dp/0470584920/ref=sr_1_2?dchild=1&keywords=Thomas+N.+Seyfried+Cancer+as+a+Metabolic+Disease&qid=1609520808&sr=8-2

Ken D. Berry, MD:
https://www.youtube.com/channel/UCIma2WOQs1Mz2AuOt6wRSUw

Paul Saladino, MD:

https://www.youtube.com/channel/UCgBg0LcHfnJD
PmFTTf677Pw

Dr. Dominic D'Agostino:
https://www.ketonutrition.org

Why Stress Spikes the Risk of Cancer:
Youtube.com/ watch?v=LAFcznRMHvM
Pr Khayat David : « L'enquête vérité : vous n'aurez
plus jamais peur du cancer », 19 septembre 2018

Yoshinori Ohsumi – Nobel Price: Molecular
Mechanisms of Autophagy in Yeast, Tokyo Institute
of Technology, 7 décembre 2016 –
publi.inserm.fr/bitstream/handle/10608/9127/MS_2
017_03_213.pdf

Vitamin K2 and cancer, Fan Xv, Jiepeng Chen, Lili
Duan, and Shuzhuang Li, juin 2018
ncbi.nlm.nih.gov/pmc/articles/PMC5958717/

Vit. D and cancer, Cedric F. Garland, Frank C. Garland,
Edward D. Gorham, Martin Lipkin, Harold Newmark,
Sharif B. Mohr, and Michael F. Holick, février 2006 –
ncbi.nlm.nih.gov/pmc/articles/PMC1470481/

Vitamin D to prevent cancer, cancer.gov, octobre
2013 – cancer.gov/about-cancer/causes-
prevention/risk/diet/vitamin-d-fact-sheet
Vitamin D cancer, cancer.gov, octobre 2013

ncbi.nlm.nih.gov/pmc/articles/PMC6074169/Cancer
terminal_impression_intérieur_17_08_21.indd

Garcinia   gummi-gutta   mskcc.org/cancer-
care/integrative-medicine/herbs/garcinia-gummi-
gutta
Honey as a natural vaccine against cancer
https://www.ncbi.nlm.nih.gov/pmc/articles/PMC394
2905/

Honey helps with cancer:
https://www.ncbi.nlm.nih.gov/pmc/articles/PMC806
9364/

Honey and cancer:
https://www.ncbi.nlm.nih.gov/pmc/articles/PMC338
5631/

> **"May food be thy medicine"**
>
> - Hippocrates

Printed in Great Britain
by Amazon

21023170R00112